For Suz …

My close friend of 40 years plus …

I've included a few with less than 3 ingredients

and no cooking just for you!

For Rebecca …

None of my cooking books,

and my historical fiction books,

and my publishing related books

would exist without your

creativity, eyes, and skills.

Inspired by one of my

favorite foodie quotes …

Health food may be good for the conscience,

but Oreos taste a hell of a lot better.

— Robert Redford

Appetizers *with* Judith

Yummy Nibbles and Starters that

WOW!

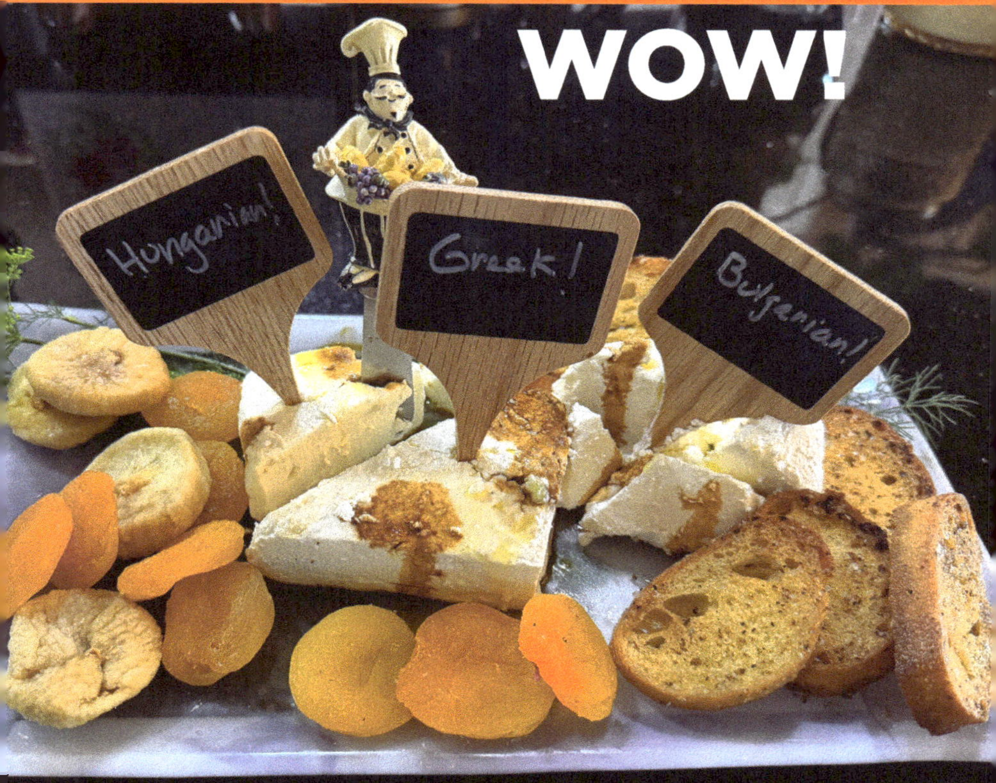

Judith Briles

MileHigh Press

Mile High Press, Ltd.
www.MileHighPress.com
MileHighPress@aol.com
303-885-4460

Appetizers with Judith
Yummy Nibbles and Starters that WOW!

Books may be purchased in quantity by contacting the publisher directly or by calling 303-885-2207.
Mile High Press, Ltd.
8122 South Quatar Circle
Aurora, Colorado 80016

Editing: Peggie Ireland, Mary Salas, Ellen Tryon
Cover and Interior Design: Rebecca Finkel, F+P Design, FPGD.com

ISBN trade KDP paperback: 978-1-885331-16-8
ISBN trade IS paperback: 978-1-959737-02-5
ISBN eBook: 978-1-885331-17-5

LCCN: 2026915867

cooking | appetizers | entertaining

contents

Welcome Back to My Kitchen

I love having friends over. Sometimes for a full meal; sometimes for a celebration; sometimes just to have nibbles and starters. And always for conversation..

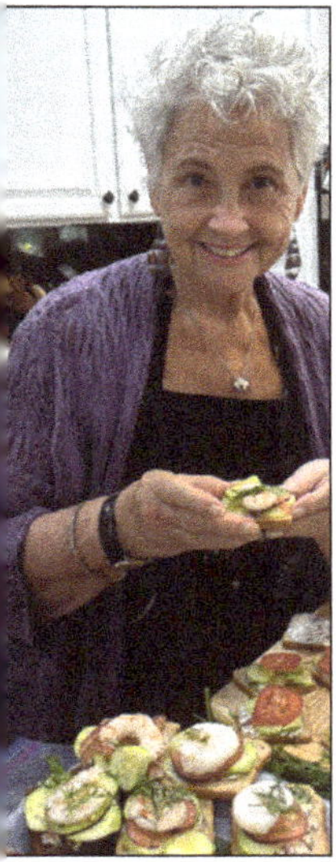

An appetizer gathering is a favorite—as a beginner, a full meal, or a spread of many. During the holidays when the house is festive, the "spread for many" that combines hot and cold offerings is my favorite.

Ten of the recipes within this book debuted at my Friend's Holiday Schmooze in 2025—the *Shrimp, Cucumber, Feta, and Dill Delights* on the cover is one of those. All became keepers and are included within—it is not uncommon for nibblers to ask if there are any leftovers.

My neighborhood in Colorado has a monthly potluck—weather is never a holdback! When I created the *South of the Border Hearty Nacho Dip Delight,* I first put it in a 9 x 13 baking dish with fresh made tortilla chips for the dipping and testing knowing that there would be a minimum of 25. Little did I know that it was to become the main course for many as my friends came back for scoop after scoop.

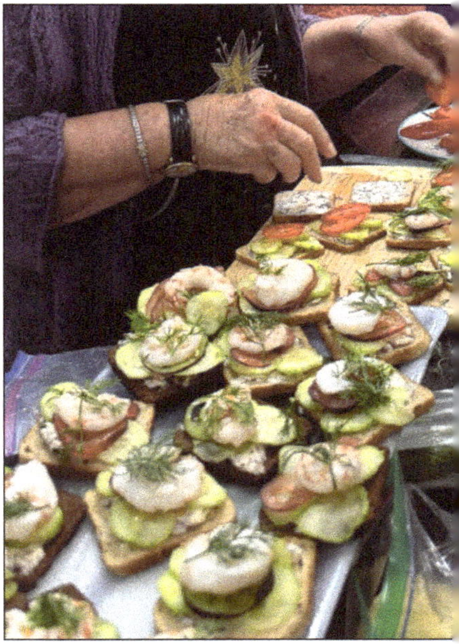

Spoiler alert: I never cook with thyme or rosemary, both I'm allergic to. I also always ask invited guests if they have allergies as well.

I love the "presentation" and setting the serving area for the season or event.

The spread of the foods for a gathering adds eye candy. As with the main dishes I create, appetizers are perfect for dabbling and playing with combining foods, herbs, and spices.

All with the objective of tasty food and great tastes. If you came to my home for a cup of sugar, I may be able to help. If you were looking for a cup of capers, I'm your gal.

Sometimes I'll call a few friends and share what I'm doing and ask if they would like to be my guinea pigs for a tasting. No one turns me down. Some of my concoctions are roaring successes … some, well, I need to tweak a tad, or let them go.

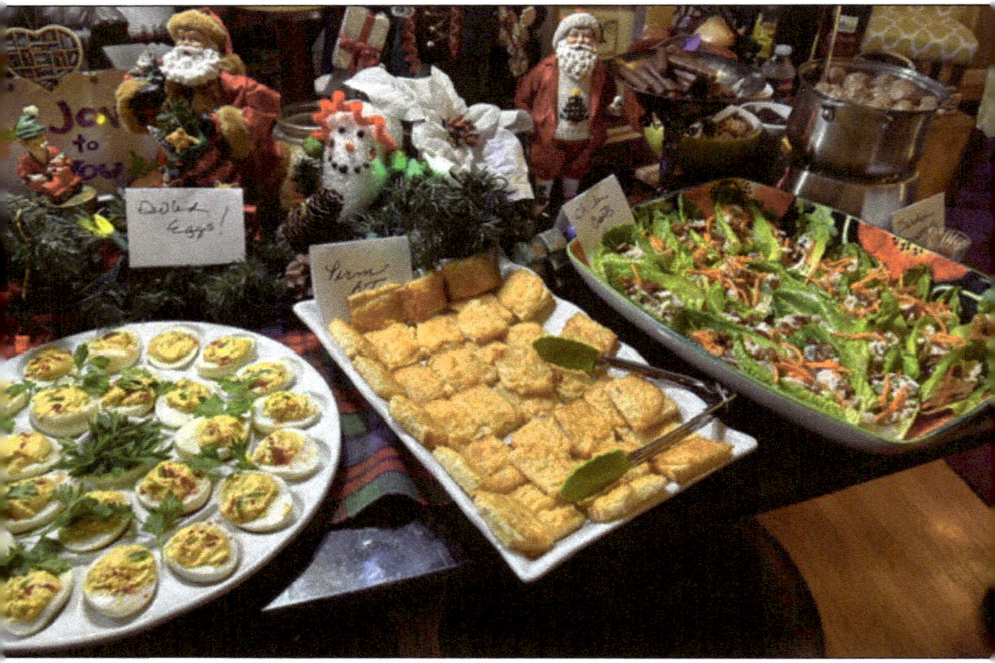

For years, friends, family, clients, staff, and visitors have asked me to share what I create. My *truthiness* is that I often just make things up as I go along, rarely making notes or writing them up. I'm a "hands-on" cook—meaning that I view other recipes as a starting point—I get to play with—always asking myself, what would I add … or remove.

It means opening the pantry or refrigerator and seeing what talks to me. And it definitely means that I don't have to go to a specialty store for exotic ingredients and that I can easily pronounce the name of an ingredient and found it in a store or quickly online.

Finally, I started to make better notes and created a separate file for each recipe.

My intention was and is not to write a cookbook with an emphasis on entertaining around dishes. I didn't want to do that, although I love entertaining around food. With friends. Both inside and outside on the deck. I share randomly on my blogs and social media when I do.

What I have for you is many of my appetizers that I rotate throughout the year. And my cheesy bite concoction is devoured as soon as it comes out of the oven.

I'm not a chef or a gourmet, but I am a cook.

Appetizers with Judith happily joins **Cooking with Judith** … and as you make them, share your photos with me. Make sure one of them has you in it, and send to my email, *Judith@Briles.com.*

Judith

Inspired by one of my

favorite foodie quotes …

"I think every woman

should have a blow torch."

— JULIA CHILD

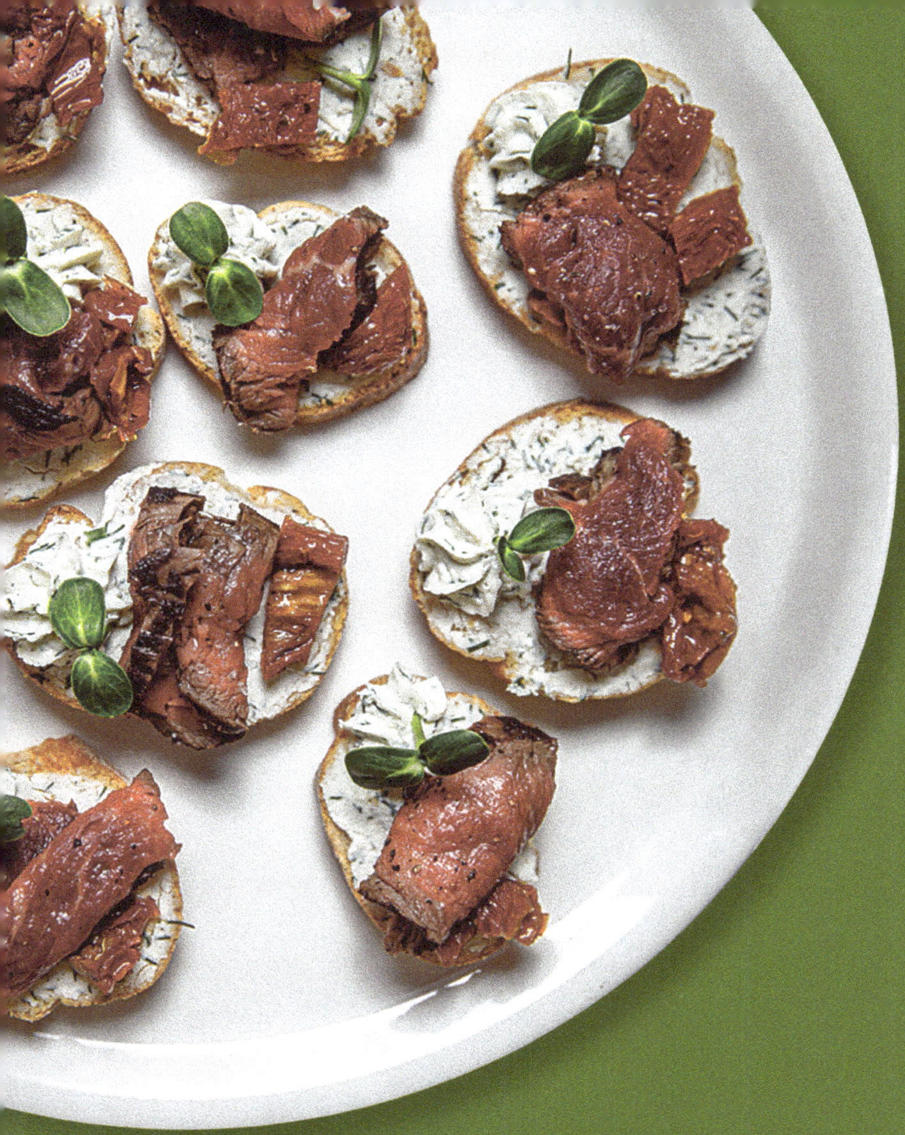

beef

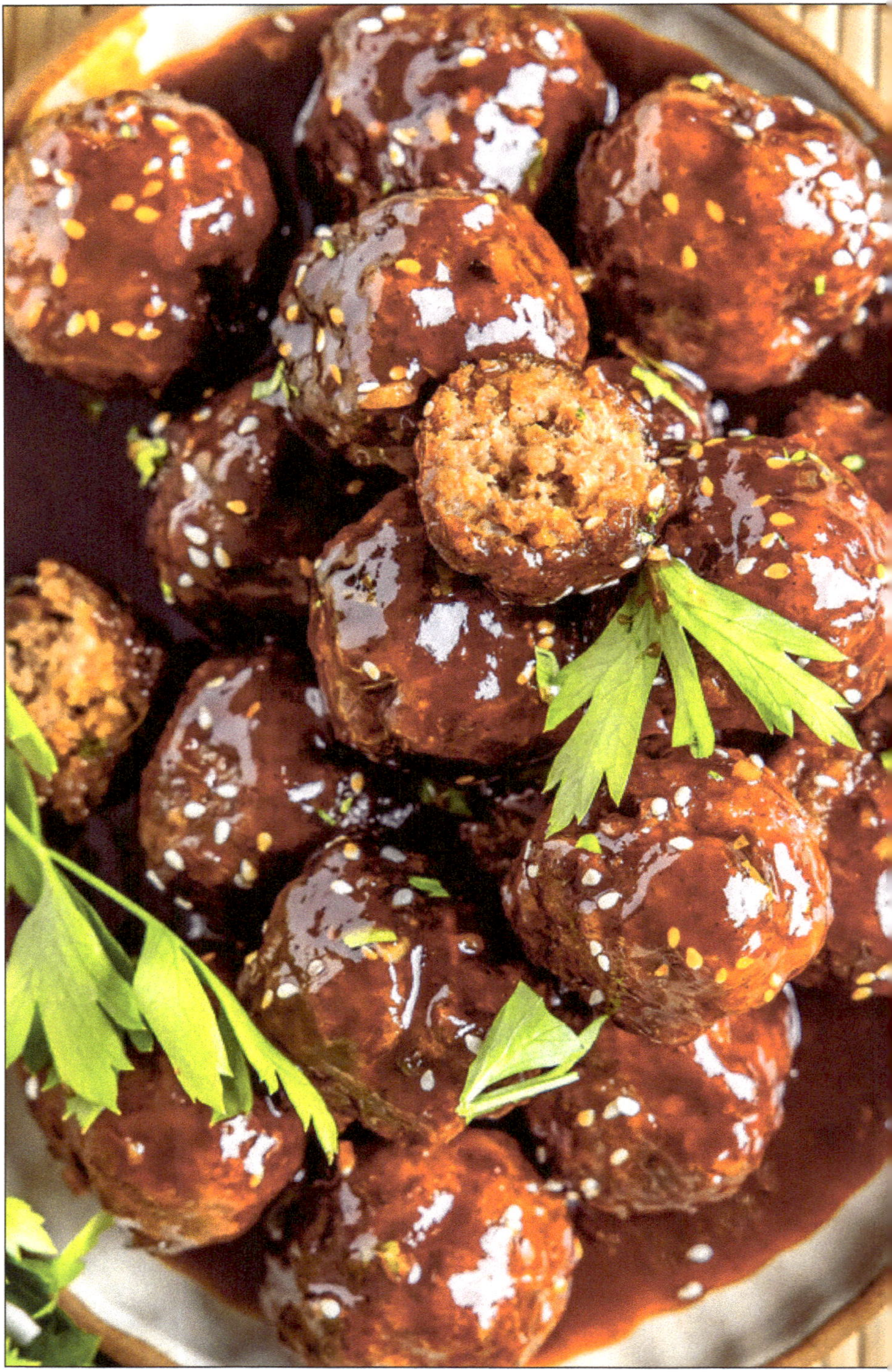

Easy Peasy Grape Meatballs

I noodled whether I wanted to include this. When I first did the grape jelly and meatball combo, I thought ... You have got to be kidding? Every host wants a no-brainer, no work, almost no-thinking snack or appetizer that will be welcomed and disappear quickly. This one is for you! It's so simple.

All ages gobbled them up. This is one that will rescue you when the OMG, they will be here in 10 minutes. That moment when: What can I fix quickly and will taste good? The one you can do almost blindfolded.

makes: 30 meatballs
prep time: 5 minutes | **heating time:** 5-10 minutes

ingredients

meatballs precooked—*I use the teriyaki with pineapple in the deli section of Costco*

12 to 18 oz jar grape jelly

Option: Sprinkle with sesame seeds. Or, or a kiss of heat, a few red pepper flakes

toothpicks

putting it all together

Use a fondue pot, a small crock pot, or even a sauce pan. Add the meatballs. Add the entire jar of grape jelly. You want enough to cover at least ¾ of the meatballs. Heat and stir. Serve with tooth-picks on the side.

Swedish Meatballs

I've been to Sweden once for a speaking engagement and sampled the Swedish Meatballs at a banquet. My taste buds wanted more.

Juicy and flavorful is how I think of Swedish Meatballs. I've done them just for John and me for dinner. Freezing the leftovers for a future meal or to add to an appetizer offering. And I've prepared for friends with all the noodle and mashed potato adds.

I eat as I cook. When I'm at the stove, I cannot reveal how many of these morsels I "consume" in the creation to the final meal. Why, oh why, don't I just include in my appetizer offerings? Why indeed.

I'm going to give you two options here. Make from scratch or do a cheat: use frozen Swedish meatballs. I get mine at the local Kroger store for under $6—with about 50 meatballs per package.

This recipe includes a savory gravy cream sauce that is to die for—I love the kiss of nutmeg and allspice. The frozen variety has a sauce, but it is lacking. Make the sauce that I have shared below. And don't forget the sour cream.

makes: 20 meatballs

prep time: 30 minutes for scratch | **cooking time:** 25 minutes

ingredients for making from scratch

1 lb ground beef, 80% lean

½ lb ground pork

2 T olive oil, divided in half—use half with mixing the meat and the other for browning meatballs.

¾ C yellow onion, finely diced

3 garlic cloves, minced

⅓ C panko breadcrumbs

⅓ C Parmesan cheese

1 large egg or 2 medium eggs, whisked

⅓ C milk

1 tsp salt

¼ tsp dried oregano

½ tsp pepper

1 tsp nutmeg

1 tsp allspice

sauce: you will use for both Scratch and Frozen versions

You will make a roux—think of it as culinary paste. I always make plenty of sauce. For the broth, I mix in Better Than Bouillon.

2 C chicken or beef broth

1 C sour cream, at room temperature

6 T butter

½ C plus 1 T flour

3 tsp Worcestershire sauce

1½ tsp Dijon mustard

2 tsp dried parsley

putting it all together

step 1: Combine the breadcrumbs, Parmesan cheese, egg, milk, onions, garlic, salt, oregano, allspice, nutmeg, and pepper. Mix with your hands to integrate all.

step 2: If frozen store-bought meatballs: Thaw..

step 3: Roll into 1½-inch meatballs and chill for 15 minutes. Overnight is okay too. Brown in batches and set aside.

continued

step 4: Make sauce. Melt butter, whisking in flour to create paste. Add the rest of the sauce ingredients. Wait until they are all merged, then add sour cream last.

Step 5: Add the meatballs back and spoon the sauce on top. Cover partially, and simmer for 10-15 minutes, or until cooked through. For frozen, they are fully cooked—you want them heated, so just let them simmer for the same about of time.

Done. *You will need toothpicks!*

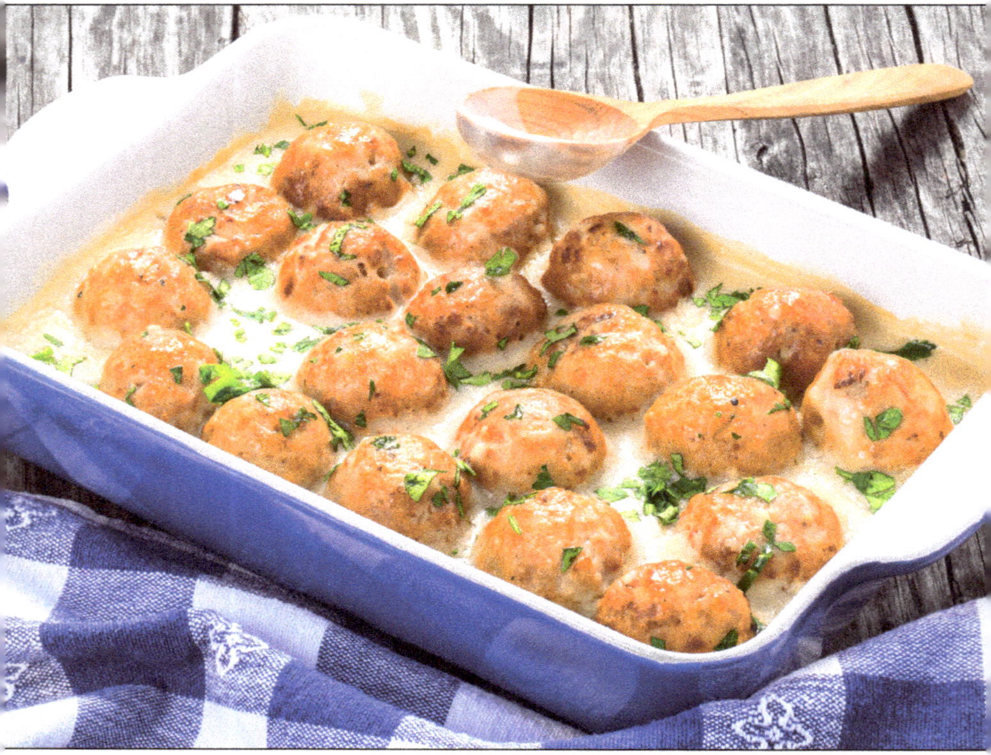

South of the Border Hearty Nacho Dip Delight

How about a comfort appetizer with a kiss of zip to it? Of course, when you add salsa, a jalapeño ranch dressing, and a little chili powder or taco seasoning, it is what you will get. This is a year-round share—either on mini plates or where guests scoop out what they want with homemade tortilla chips (my favorite), store bought tortilla chips (your choice), or Fritos Scoops. Heck, I've even added it to a cooked taco shell with a fringe of lettuce on top when the taco craving taste buds surface! When I first served this, the crowd came back for seconds and thirds.

What I like about this dip is that I usually have all the ingredients in my pantry and/or freezer.

makes: 10 to 12 cups—*it's huge!*
prep time: 15 minutes | **cooking time:** 25 minutes at 350°F

ingredients

- 1 lb ground beef
- 1 onion, chopped
- 1 15.5 oz can of black beans (drained)
- 1 16 oz can of refried beans
- 1½ C chunky salsa
- 1 (10 oz) can whole kernel corn, drained
- ¾ C black olives, sliced
- ¾ C green olives, sliced
- 1 C creamy salad dressing … *jalapeño ranch or sour cream*
- 1 tsp chili powder or ½ packet taco seasoning *I like Trader Joe's*
- 2 C crushed tortilla chips (your choice) or mix with Fritos
- 2 C cheese … Colby, Mexican mix, Jack, one or mix them up

continued

Serve large chips—the ones you buy in a bag … or quickly fry up tortillas that have been cut into pieces and add your homemade touch. I suggest you lightly salt these when you remove them from cooking before oil dries.

putting it all together

step 1: Sauté onion with ground beef. Mix in chili powder or taco seasoning.

step 2: In a 9x13 baking dish, make layers:
Beef mixture first on the bottom, then spread the beans, corn, salsa, salad dressing/sour cream, chips, and the cheese on top

step 3: Bake for 25 minutes … and definitely serve hot!

Have extra-large tortilla chips or Frito Scoops for the dip. And add dip to the concoction on a small plate that includes other appetizers. Make sure you have forks available.

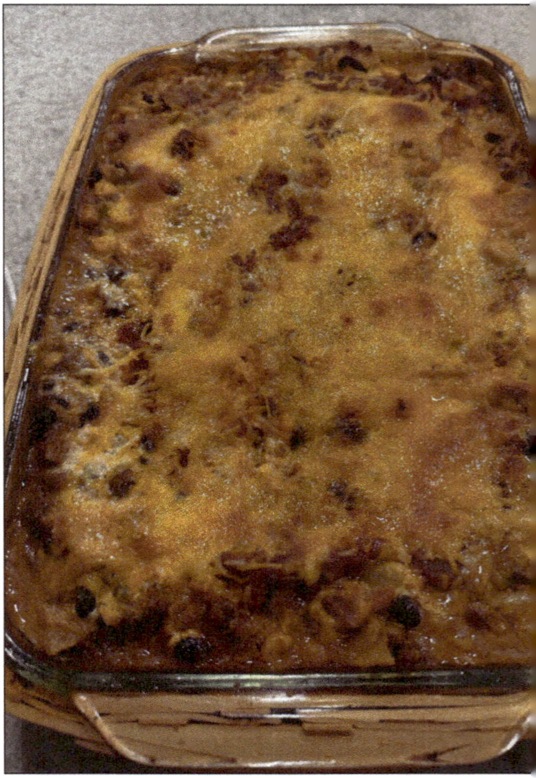

Steak Bites

Tasty bite-sized beef is usually popular with a crowd. Whether broiled or barbecued, they will disappear quickly. Always serve from warm to sizzling, for a medium-cooked outcome. It's the marinade that enhances the juiciness and taste. Marinate up to 2 hours for sirloin and strip steaks. Flank steaks need more time—up to 4 hours. I eat little beef, but I always serve it in an appetizer array.

Steak Bites, with the marinade I use for dishes that enhance anything south of the border, are yummy and a stand-alone. If you are a "dip" person, you can always add your favorite dip or two in a small bowl for your guests. A creamy horseradish or a bearnaise is a good add.

makes: 12 to 20 Bites
grill or broil | **prep time:** 20 minutes outside of marinade time
cooking time: 6-8 minutes

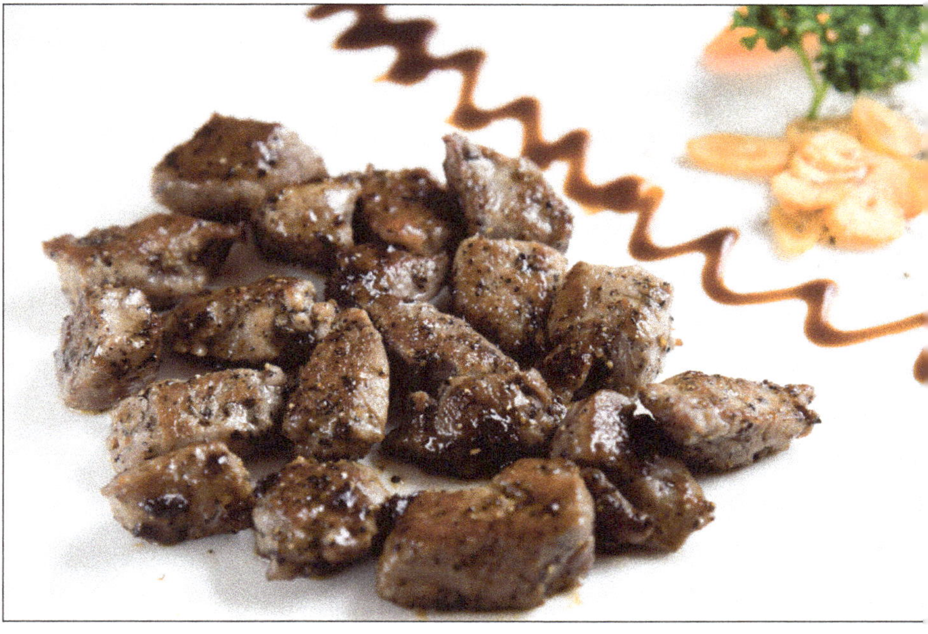

ingredients

steak, 2 lbs or less … *Your choice: sirloin, strip, or flank. Plan on bite-sized pieces no bigger than one inch.*

marinade

¾ C olive oil

5 T tarragon vinegar

1 C orange juice or ½ C orange sauce

1 C cilantro

2 limes, juiced

1 lemon, juiced

5 garlic cloves, minced

1 tsp cumin

1 tsp salt

putting it all together

step 1: Mix all marinade ingredients. Either place the steak in a dish to cover or add it to a zippered storage bag with the marinade. Make sure you turn it a few times during the marinade process.

step 2: Broil or grill your steak to the desired temp—medium is usually safe and flavorful. When cooking steak, add marinade to keep it moist. Broil or grill for 3 to 4 minutes each side, and let it rest for 5 to 10 minutes. Remove the steak from the heat when it reaches 125°F–130°F.

step 3: Cut into bite-sized pieces and serve immediately with toothpicks on a platter or a server to scoop up the amount your guests want—rarely one!

If you are adding a sauce, have it ready in small bowls with a spoon.

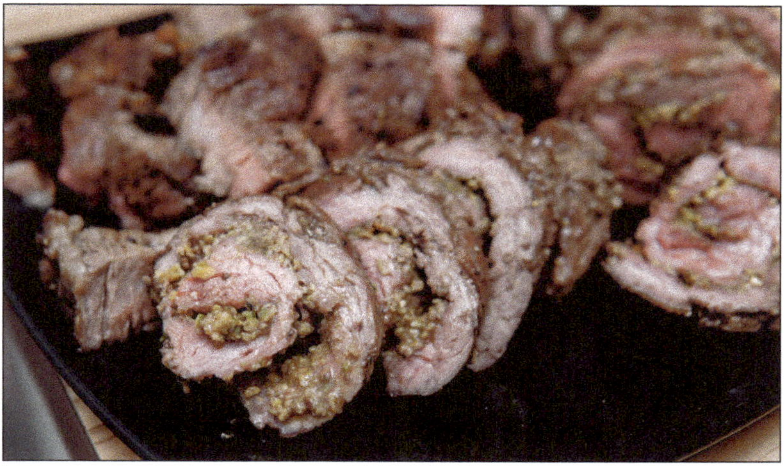

Steak and Mushroom Wheelies

Flank steak can be versatile in your appetizer offerings. How about adding mushrooms to your steak that will be cut to wheelies that you have marinated the steak in. Prepare the mushroom stuffing you have created and spread it on top of the steak. You will roll it tightly. Cooking does not take long. Let it rest for 5-10 minutes after removing from the oven, then slice your wheelies into quarter-inch slivers. You could do another add, such as a creamy sauce to dip in. I'm thinking horseradish.

The pinwheels are easily made by slicing the cooked flank steak after it is cooked.

Rolled flank steak takes longer to cook. Searing the steak for a few minutes before placing in the oven will reduce your cooking time by about 10 minutes. I use a cast iron skillet for the searing and baking—all in one.

makes: 15 wheelies | **preheat oven:** to 375°F
marinate time: 2 to 3 hours | **prep time:** 15 minutes
sear time: 8 minutes | **cooking time:** 25-35 minutes
resting time: 5 minutes

ingredients

2–2½ lbs flank steak

3 green onions, roughly chopped, plus more for garnish if desired

½ C soy sauce

½ C vegetable oil

2 garlic cloves, minced

2 T honey

2 T apple cider vinegar or white vinegar

ingredients mushroom stuffing

4 mushrooms of each: sliced cremini, shiitake, and baby portobello

1 Vidalia onion, finely chopped

1 T olive oil

1 T butter, melted

4 garlic cloves, minced

½ tsp salt

½ tsp black pepper

Gently clean mushrooms and cut stems. Mix all ingredients.

putting it all together

step 1: Create your marinade. Add green onions, soy sauce, vegetable oil, garlic, honey, and vinegar. Mix well and pour the marinade over the steak. Place in a zippered storage bag and press any extra air from the bag and seal. Refrigerate for 2-3 hours.

step 2: Combine all ingredients for mushroom stuffing. Set aside.

step 3: Remove steak from marinade and bring to room temperature. Spread the mushroom stuffing on top of it. Roll tightly and secure the roll with a string.

step 4: optional, but recommended: Rolled flank steak takes longer to cook. Searing the steak for a few minutes before placing in the oven will reduce your cooking time by about 10 minutes. Heat a little oil in a heavy, oven-safe skillet over high heat and sear the rolled steak on all sides for 1–2 minutes per side to build a crust and encase in the stuffing.

step 5: Transfer the skillet to a preheated oven (between 350°F and 375°F) and bake for 20-40 minutes, depending on your target internal temperature of 130°F to 135°F.

step 6: Remove the skillet from oven and let meat rest for 5 minutes. Remove string. With a sharp knife, slice into ⅛ to ¼ inch slices. If needed, secure pinwheels with toothpicks.

step 7: Transfer cooked pinwheels to a serving platter and keep warm. Serve drizzled with any juices that have accumulated on the platter with a smidge of salt and pepper. Include the **Creamy Horseradish Sauce** for dipping.

Creamy Horseradish Sauce

In a few minutes and four ingredients (plus salt/pepper), this sauce adds a bold, feisty flavor for dipping pleasure and is ideal for meats.

makes: 1 cup | **prep time:** 5 miutes

ingredients

- 1 C sour cream
- 2½ to 3 T prepared horseradish
- 1 tsp Dijon mustard
- 1 tsp fresh lemon juice
- 1 tsp kosher salt
- ground black pepper as desired

putting it all together

In a medium bowl, combine all ingredients and whisk. Chill before serving.

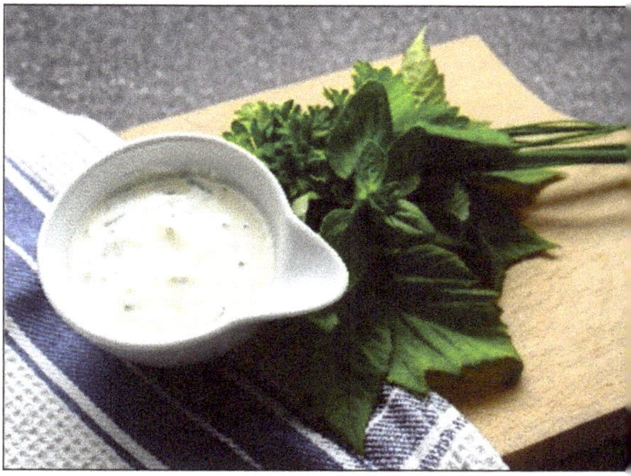

Marinated Flank Steak Crostini

I promise—my marinated flank steak crostini will be a hit when you serve them. They are easily made by slicing flank steak thin and marinating for a few hours in a very simple marinade. Flank steak cooks quickly, 4 minutes per side.

makes: 20 to 30 crostini
broil: 500 °F
marinate time: 2-3 hours | **prep time:** 10 minutes
broil: approximately 6-8 minutes until internal temp is 135°F
rest time: 5 minutes

ingredients

2–2½ lb flank steak

3 green onions, roughly chopped, plus more for garnish if desired

½ C soy sauce

½ C vegetable oil

2 garlic cloves, minced

2 T honey

2 T apple cider vinegar or white vinegar

small jar sun-dried tomatoes

option: Asparagus, pencil thin

baguette, sliced ⅛ to ¼ inch thick

horseradish sauce

putting it all together

step 1: Create your marinade. Add green onions, soy sauce, vegetable oil, garlic, honey, and vinegar to a blender or food processor and blend until well combined. Pour marinade over steak. Press any extra air from the bag and seal. Refrigerate for two hours.

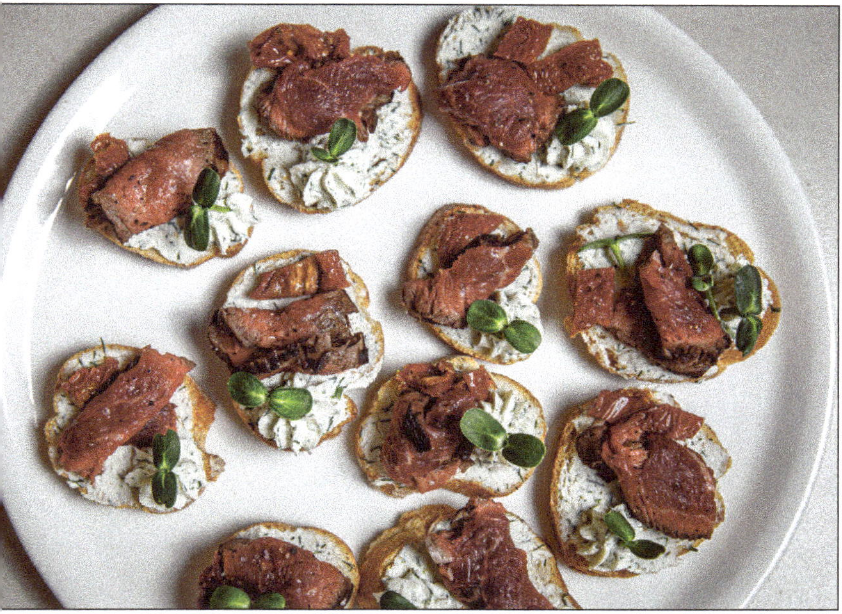

step 2: Remove steak strips from the bag and discard leftover marinade. Broil until meat temp is between 130°F to 135°F. Slice the flank steak across and against the grain into ¼-inch thick slices and place the slices into a large zippered bag bag.

step 3: Slice baguette. Make **Crostini,** see page 45.

step 4: Assemble your crostini. Spread **Horseradish Sauce,** see page 13, on top of crostini. Add a sliver of cooked flank steak, sun-dried tomatoes, and, if you have, one or two asparagus pieces.

Seize the moment ...
Remember all those women
on the 'Titanic' who waved off
the dessert cart.

— Erma Bombeck

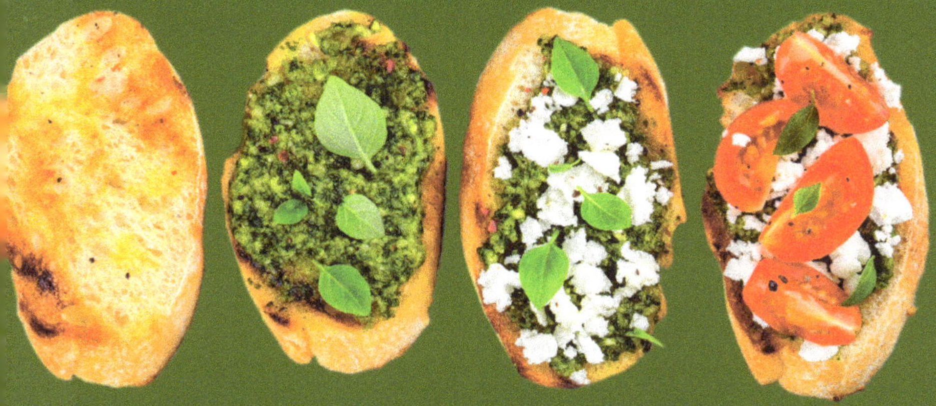

charcuterie board

Croutons … Take Away Munchies

I love fresh croutons in my leaf salads. I dislike any that come from the pre-packaged versions available in every grocery store. For years beyond my recall, I've been making my own, easy peasy croutons to add to salads and soups. Routinely when I'm in a grocery store, I head to the section where the bread is placed once it is pulled from the shelves. Perfect … the first ingredient. All that is needed to be added is olive oil, garlic salt, a kiss of pepper and voilà …the oven beckons to start the mouth-popping party!

And that's where the munchies come in. There has never been a time when I haven't done my own tasting when they come out—never. And it's not just one or two. Nope, I can eat ten plus. One of my friends asked if I would make a batch for her birthday present. I've had friends leave after a dinner party, asking for a drive home baggie … that they consume on the way home.

Although sourdough bread is my preferred choice, I discovered that the breadsticks at my local Olive Garden restaurant work as a quick substitute. Once I tested the uneaten ones when returning home from an evening meal, my light bulb when off—these sticks cut up are the perfect size for croutons. The folks at Olive Garden always bring extras when I ask for them to take home with me.

Crouton Munchies … why not have a bowl for nibblers?

makes: 5 to 6 cups | **preheat:** oven to 375°F
prep time: 10 minutes | **cooking time:** 10 minutes

ingredients

1 loaf of bread—*day old sourdough has better density than French Bread; a baguette cut up works well, too.*

½ C olive oil

6 T Parmesan cheese, grated

¾ tsp garlic salt

½ tsp black pepper

putting it all together

step 1: Cut your loaf in cubes of less than one inch—small pieces, ¾ inch. Perfection cutting not needed.

step 2: Use a large baking sheet and generously spread olive oil on it. Shake garlic salt and pepper on the oil and mix with a small spatula or your fingers. Add the bread cubes and mix your baking sheet ingredients with your hands to coat all sides. Sprinkle Parmesan cheese and quickly mix with uncooked croutons.

step 3: Bake until a light golden brown.

step 4: Remove from oven and place on paper towels to absorb any excess oil. When cool, add to multiple quart size zippered storage bags. Some for immediate use, some for freezing.

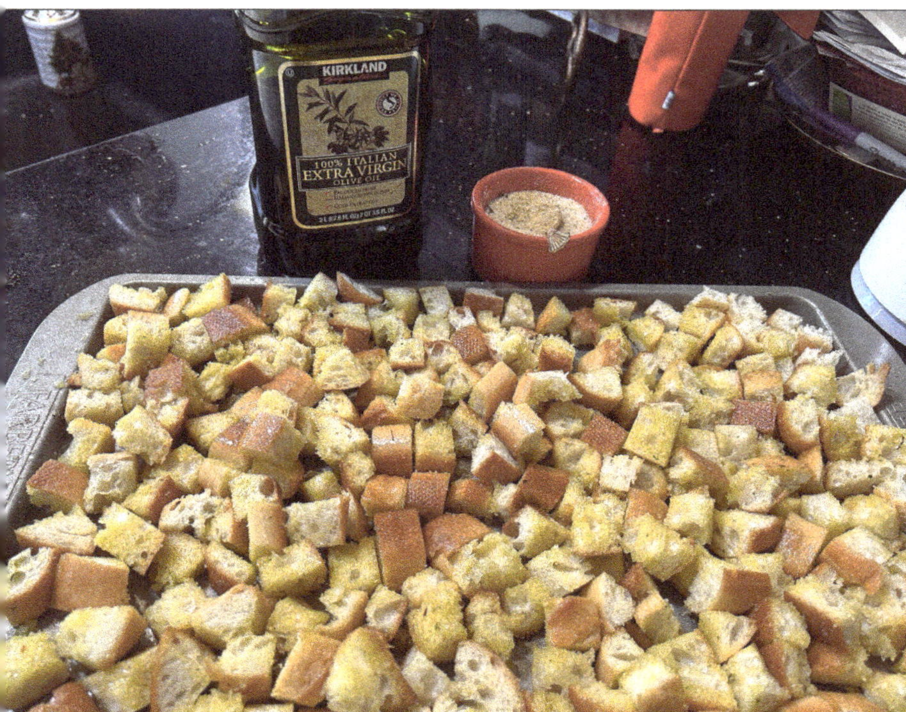

Feta Cheese Tasting from Abroad

I'm a fan of a rich, creamy feta cheese, and the best I've found comes from Europe. A much creamier one than its American cousin and what you usually find in a lettuce salad.

Think France, Hungary, Bulgaria, Greece. I find mine at Middle Eastern grocery stores. Make yours a Feta Tasting. You could add a fourth cheese, an American feta, and let let your guests do a comparison taste. Add olive oil and balsamic vinegar to dribble over for your guests to nibble over the feta concoction. Dry apricots and a variety of olives are a welcome addition. You might want to take a few whole heads of garlic and bake—cutting the tips off and letting your guests spread the softened baked garlic clove on a cracker or crostini.

Serve with artisan crackers, crostini, and a fresh sliced baguette —warmed is always welcome. Choices for all ....

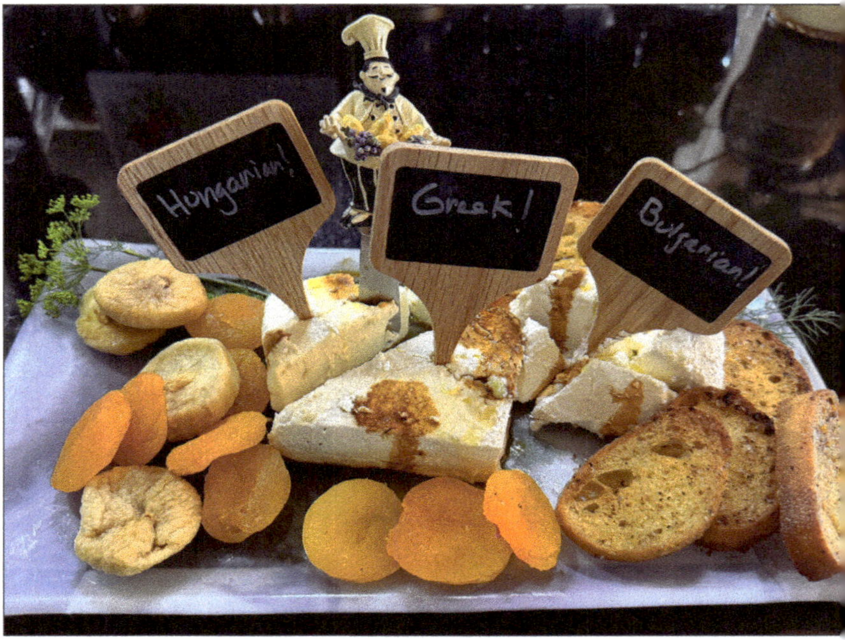

servings: 6 to 20, depending on how much cheese you display
prep time: 15 minutes | **cooking time:** none

ingredients

feta cheese ¼ to ½ lb each – at least three European … plus one American

olive oil

balsamic vinegar

½ lb of dried apricots—*add your choice of other dried fruits*

olives—Kalamata, green with stuffing (garlic-jalapeño-bleu cheese)

artisan crackers and baguette, sliced

putting it all together

Remember … cheeses need to be served at room temperature. I take mine out of the refrigerator 30–60 minutes before guests arrive and set up my presentation tray.

Baguette—slice … you can offer fresh or some that have been baked slightly. My preference is just sliced. Each slice absorbs the olive oil and the kiss of balsamic vinegar.

If you are making crostini, bake per my **Crostini** recipe on page 45.

French Onion Baked Brie WOW

Hello caramelized onions, a welcome addition and surprise to your guests. Add your favorite artisan crackers, baguette slices, or crostini that have been lightly baked. As I write this, I can already taste it. Yum!

Brie can usually be found at a late afternoon gathering or early evening. I love topping it with favorite things. Sometimes, topped with jams—blackberry, raspberry, marionberry, even fig. Other times, baking with a favorite topping wrapped in puff pastry or phyllo dough. Why not, I thought, just let the warmed cheese do its "ooze thing" … why not indeed!

When you are serving an appetizer with baked cheese in it … assume that it is meant to be warm with the first bite. Meaning that you don't pull it from the refrigerator as the doorbell rings. I'm a fan

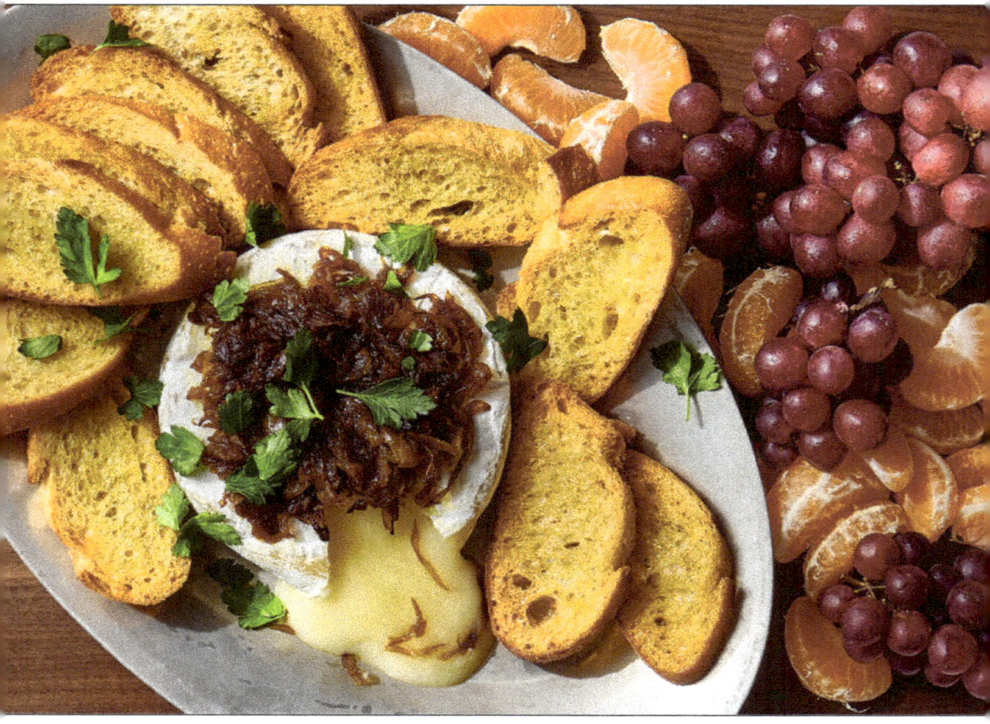

of a tangy Brie or the more subtle Camembert. Your presentation will add a caramelized onion topping to it. Your guests will make the first cut in the baked cheese round and cheese will ooze out, ready to fill your apple, bread, crostini, sliced baguette, or cracker accompaniment.

The caramelized onions can be prepared the day before and stored to use later if you choose … or make them before you bake the Brie or Camembert, just piling them on top before the two go into the oven together. Bake and serve.

makes: 6 to 10 servings
preheat: oven to 350°F
prep time: 10-15 minutes | **cooking time:** 40 minutes

ingredients

2-3 T olive oil or butter

1 tsp balsamic vinegar to taste

1 tsp sugar

½ tsp pepper—*sometimes I add lemon pepper as well*

salt—a pinch

1 large onion—Spanish, Walla Walla, Vidalia— thinly sliced

Brie round (at least 8 oz)—*don't remove the rind*

baguette, sliced—*sliced as is or lightly toasted. Or* **Crostini** *on page 45*

Artisan crackers of choice

Chopped fresh herbs, such as dill, parsley, mint, or chives

Adds for your serving platter: dried apricots, seedless grapes, seedless mandarin oranges (Cuties), and your favorite nuts. *Visual and tasty fun.*

putting it all together

step 1: In a skillet, heat olive oil or butter over medium heat—add sliced onion, salt, pepper, and sugar. Cook until edges are browned, for about 25 minutes. If it looks dry, add a tablespoon of water. You want your onions to get jammy. Add balsamic vinegar and another pinch of salt, if needed. Tip … you can do your onions a day ahead.

step 2: Slice your baguette. I usually plan on freezing my unused slices for another time. If you are making crostini, brush with olive oil, and sprinkle a little garlic powder or Parmesan cheese on top. Bake 5 to 7 minutes. *Tip … I make plenty of these and use in salads as substitute croutons.*

step 3: Place your Brie in a ceramic baking dish and pile the onion mix on top. Bake for approximately 10 minutes or until the cheese begins to ooze.

step 4: Serve at once with your crostini, sliced baguette, and/or artisan crackers.

Garlic Nuts

What is a gathering without a bowl of nuts of some sort? These are one of my favorites—mixed nuts with lots of garlic and Parmesan. The truffle seasoning is the surprise, as are garlic cloves in my bowl of nuts. Instead of the more pungent taste, the baking breaks them down. If you are not a fan of peeling cloves, the cheat I use when I need lots of garlic is to get the packs of peeled garlic. Your max time of prepping and cooking is reduced to 20 minutes.

makes: 2 cups—*they will go fast!*
preheat oven: 350°F
prep time: 20 minutes | **cooking time:** 20 minutes

ingredients

4 garlic heads or Costco's Garland Organic Peeled Garlic

2 C unsalted mixed nuts

4 tsp olive oil

1½ tsp Truffle Parmesan & Black Garlic Seasoning—
I get this at Costco or Trader Joe's

putting it all together

Peel all the cloves of garlic (approximately 40) OR remove from packaging that contains peeled cloves. Mix with Truffle Parmesan and Black Garlic Seasoning and olive oil. On a baking sheet, roast for 15 minutes or until garlic softens and is a golden color.

Mix quickly with your nuts and roast another 5 minutes. Put in a small serving bowl with a dipper-type spoon for your guests to serve themselves.

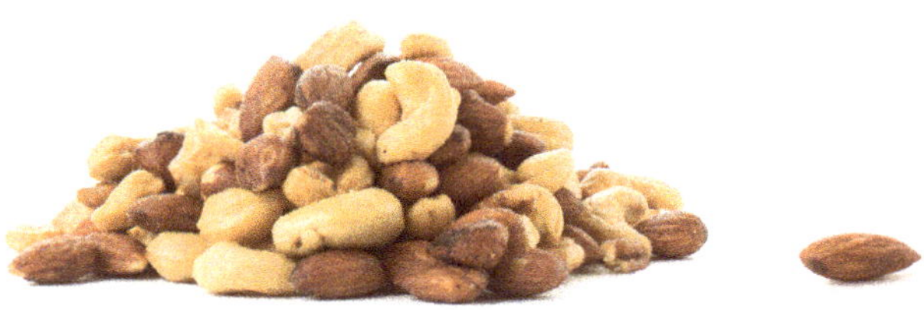

Greek Salad Skewers

makes: 20 skewers

prep time: 30 minutes | **cooking time:** none

ingredients

½ English cucumber, cut in bite-size chunks

kosher salt and freshly ground black pepper

Feta cheese, cut into small cubes – *if you can get a Bulgarian, French, Greek, or Hungarian feta, use instead—find at a Middle Eastern grocer … so much better than American. Otherwise, get a block or thick sliced*

pitted Kalamata olives, whole

small ripe tomatoes, halved

extra virgin olive oil and/or balsamic vinegar to drizzle

optional adds
artichoke hearts, halved; red or yellow bell peppers, roasted, halved; basil, finely chopped to sprinkle on top

skewers

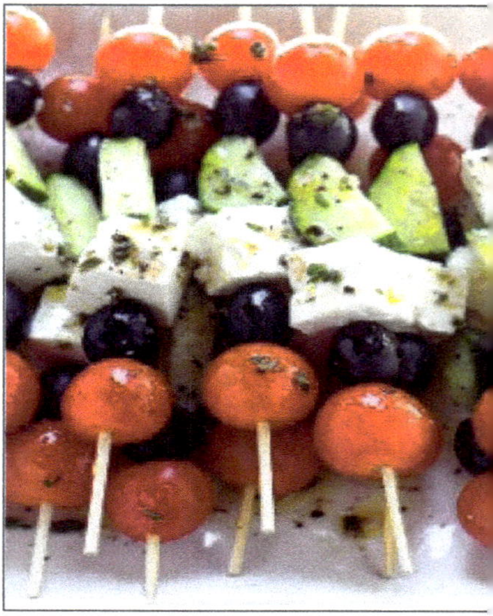

putting it all together

step 1: Salt your cucumber chunks. Place in a colander and let the excess water drip for about 30 minutes. Remove and gently rinse salt. Pat dry.

step 2: Make layers on your skewer with cucumber, artichoke, olives, peppers, feta cheese, and tomatoes on ends. Drizzle with a smidge of olive oil, sprinkle with black pepper and basil leaves. Serve.

Onion Dip with Sweet Chili Swizzle

Onion dips and their variations are always a dipping favorite. Onion is one of my favorites, and adding a condiment to complement brings out the yum factor. Sometimes dips are smooth; sometimes with bits; and other times with easily identified onion pieces. It's a choice. One of mine is a sweet chili sauce. Experiment with it. I think you will enjoy it.

makes: 2 cups

prep time: 10 minutes | **cooking time:** 15 minutes

ingredients

- 2 large onions, yellow or Vidalia
- 4 T butter, unsalted
- 4 T olive oil
- 2 T sweet chili sauce
- 1 tsp kosher salt
- 1½ tsp onion powder
- ½ tsp sugar
- 1 tsp apple cider vinegar
- 1 tsp black pepper (freshly ground is best)
- ½ C (4 oz) cream cheese
- 16 oz sour cream
- chives or parsley for garnish (optional)
- "heavy" chip and cracker favorites for spreading

putting it all together

step 1: Peel and slice onions. Depending on the size of the onions, you will have two to three cups.

step 2: Melt butter with oil in a large pan over medium heat. Sauté onions, salt and pepper for 10 minutes. Reduce the heat and cook for another 15-20 minutes to caramelize and turn golden brown.

Add in the onion powder, sugar, and apple cider vinegar. Continue to cook, uncovered, stirring every 1-2 minutes until the onions have turned a deep golden brown.

step 3: Let cool on the stove for about 10 minutes.

step 4: Blend cream cheese and sour cream until smooth. Add in sweet chili sauce. Stir in onions and mix all well. Taste for season adjustments. Garnish with chives or parsley.

step 5: Serve at room temperature with chips, naan, and baguette slices.

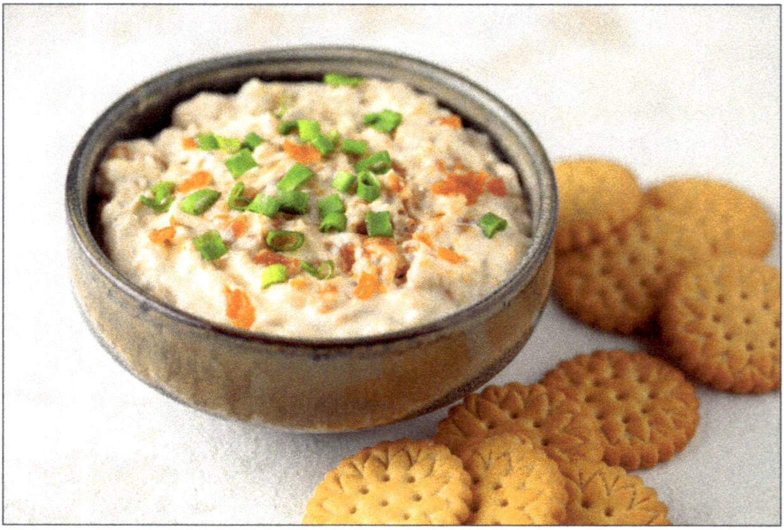

Pistachio Cheese Lollipops

These lollipops are always a fun, visual delight to your guests. They are different and easy peasy to create and display. You want a cheese that you can mold/shape quickly around the grape center surprise inside. Make sure you use seedless grapes … red or green. Why not mix it up?

If you can get a Roquefort that doesn't crumble quickly, use it. Goat cheese always works. Make sure you pull out your cheese from the refrigerator 30 minutes before you shape it for ease, then refrigerate after rolling in the pistachios … again, pulling it out about 30 minutes before your guests are expected … you don't want cheese served chilly.

makes: 20 lollipops | **prep time:** 30 minutes | **cooking time:** none

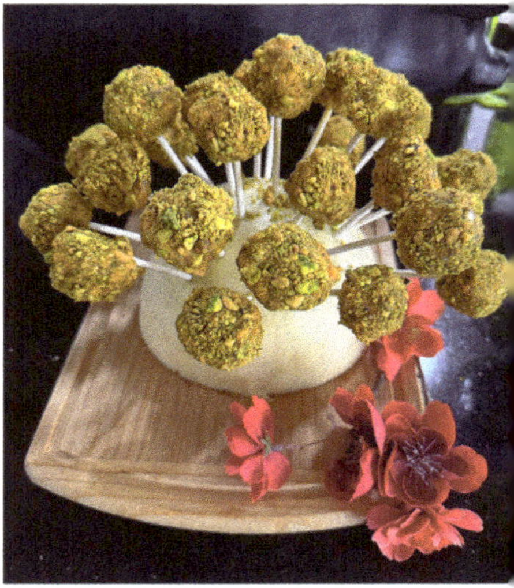

ingredients

1 goat cheese log … *or you can substitute in Roquefort, Cabrales or Stilton cheese*

Red and/or green seedless grapes, large

Pistachios, chop small or grind … get salted and roasted

Sesame seeds-toasted (optional)

putting it all together

step 1: Depending on how many you do, plan on 30 minutes for wrapping around the grape and shaping cheese over each to cover. Then roll in the pistachio mix.

step 2: One grape at a time, shape the balls with your hands around the grape so that it is fully encased—*that's the surprise.*

step 3: Roll cheese ball in crushed pistachios or toasted sesame seeds. Use a mini skewer to poke on one side of your cheese ball.

For display, stand upright in mini glass or ceramic container … or take a honeydew melon half and poke in skewers or cake pop sticks.

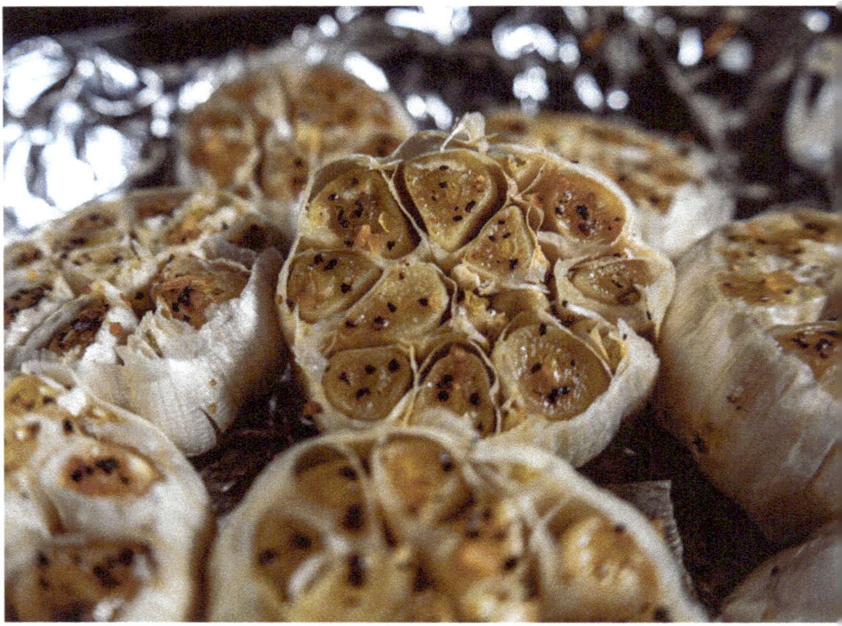

Roasted Garlic Heads

This is a fun appetizer that is unexpected. Each summer, my friend, Connie gathers up a variety of garlic heads. She bakes … We gather … taste … definitely enjoy … and then rank which is the best. The surprise is always the emerging of a slight sweetness of the garlic in its transformation from raw to roasted. Yum! Perfect for a gathering of 8. Make sure you have your favorite appetizer beverage—this is a fun conversation starter.

makes: each garlic head = 10 cooked cloves; plan on 2-3 cloves for each serving | **preheat:** oven to 400°F | **prep time:** 5 minutes
cooking time: 45 minutes

ingredients

- garlic heads
- olive oil
- pepper
- artisan crackers
- baguette, sliced
- aluminum foil

putting it all together

step 1: Remove all but one layer of the loose papery skin from the outside of the garlic bulb, leaving the entire bulb intact. Next, cut off the top of the bulb. You want to leave the top portions of the cloves exposed and peeking through.

step 2: Place the garlic bulb, cut side up, on foil. Typically, I use two squares for each head. Drizzle the olive oil over the top of the bulb, then rub the entire bulb skin with the oil.

step 3: Form a loose foil wrapping around the garlic and crimp the edges to seal.

step 4: Roast for 45 minutes in a small baking dish or on a baking sheet. Do a test to see if the garlic is cooked. Unwrap one of the foils and insert a small, sharp knife. If soft, you are done. If not, roast a few more minutes, 5 to 10.

Types of Garlic

hardneck garlic: is easy to peel and most often found at your local grocery store. Shelf life is a few months. Common varieties include: Rocambole, Chesnok Red, German White, Polish Hardneck, Persian Star, Purple Stripe, Porcelain

There are so many names to get your attention. Harvesting starts as early as March and as late as December.

Baja California white: bright white cloves; bold garlic flavor; harvested in June.

California white: papery skin with creamy white cloves; spicy flavor; harvested in June.

Chinese white: light gold to white color with crescent cloves; creamy and pungent; harvested in June.

Mexican purple: porcelain & purple color with large cloves; spicy when raw but milder once cooked; harvested in March.

Argentina white: white/cream color; strong taste; harvested in December.

softneck garlic: looks different from Hardneck varieties. Sometimes you will find this on braid hanging in a store or farmer's market. The skin is hard to peel, giving them a longer shelf life than hardneck garlic. There are two main varieties: Silverskin and Artichoke

Spicy Popcorn

Rarely do I see popcorn as an appetizer offering … and why not? Nuts of some sort are usually in the mix. Popcorn will catch your guests' attention, and this one has a bit of a kick to it. DO NOT use microwave popcorn. For me, it's all about the taste and experience.

makes: one large bowl
prep time: 3 minutes | **cooking time:** a few minutes, until popped

ingredients

3½ oz popcorn

2 T canola or vegetable oil

½ tsp salt

4 T butter

½ tsp paprika

¼ tsp chili powder or Tajin seasoning

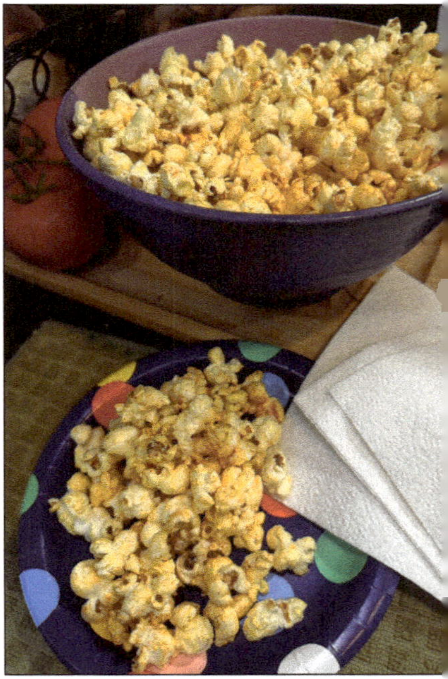

putting it all together

Add canola or vegetable oil to a large pot. Add corn kernels and spread out. Cover with a lid over medium-high heat. When popping starts, shake the pot. This all happens in a few minutes.

Move into a large bowl and drizzle with butter. Add salt, paprika, and chili powder or Tajin and TOSS. Mix and serve in a bowl with a large scooping spoon.

Tasty Parmesan Bites

A crowd pleaser and easy peasy are what these nibbles are. They disappear as soon as they come out of the oven. When I can, I quickly move them to a platter and let my crowd know. Better yet, I will often move amongst them if I have a large gathering to say hello and be the "waitress" with the platter in my offering hands.

The ingredients are beyond simple—white bread with crusts removed, mayonnaise, minced garlic, and lots of Parmesan cheese. That's it. If you love garlic, add more. You can also use garlic powder.

I've served these at Teas I've hosted ... with soup ... with salad ... with drinks and schmoozing on my deck in the afternoon with friends.

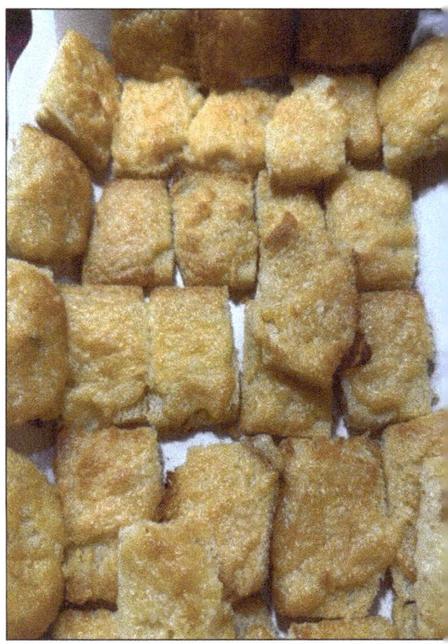

makes: 20 to 25 bites
preheat oven: 350°F
prep time: 10 minutes
cooking time: 6 minutes or less

ingredients

- 1 loaf of white bread, crusts removed
- 1 C mayonnaise
- 1 C Parmesan cheese, grated
- 2-3 garlic cloves, minced

putting it all together

step 1: Remove the crusts from the bread and cut each slice into four pieces.

step 2: Mince garlic. Add to the mayonnaise and Parmesan cheese and mix all together. Generously spread on top of each small piece of bread.

step 3: Place on a baking sheet and bake until you see a slight bubbling appear and the top starts turning a golden hue on top of each piece. Serve immediately.

Twisted Garlic Knots

When I'm cooking with garlic, I love the aroma in the kitchen area. Someone walks through my front door, the first thing they say, "It smells good in here ...." These are ideal as munchie appetizers or as an add to a salad or soup offering. These go in the oven within 20 minutes of serving them. And DO NOT microwave.

makes: 10 knots | **preheat:** oven 350°F | **prep time:** 15 minutes **cooking time:** will range from 15-20 minutes. High altitudes will need to add one or two minutes.

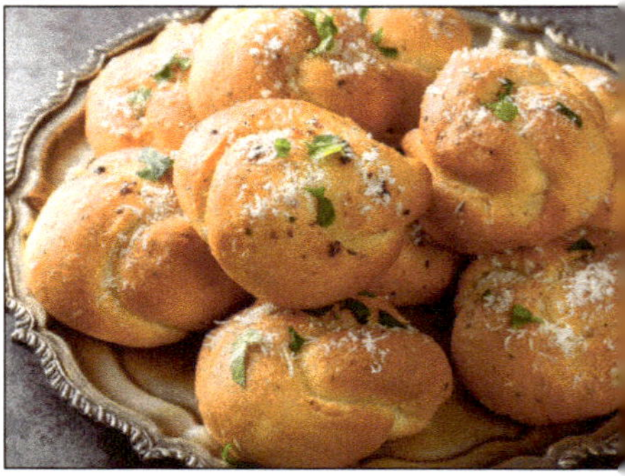

ingredients

8 oz pizza dough—store bought

½ to ¾ C Parmesan cheese

5 garlic cloves

basil or parsley, finely chopped

3 T butter

sea salt for sprinkling when knots come out of the oven

putting it all together

step 1: You want your baking sheet to be lightly oiled to place each knot on.

step 2: Roll out the pizza dough and cut it into strips that are eight inches long. Tie the strips into a simple knot. Bake.

step 3: Mince garlic. Melt the butter, adding the garlic, and sauté until the garlic is a light toasty color. Keep warm, and when the knots come out of the oven, roll them in the mixture.

step 4: Sprinkle with a little sea salt, Parmesan cheese, and a smidge of parsley or basil immediately out of oven and serve.

Whipped Feta Dip

Party time always welcomes dips. Why not add a super creamy Whipped Feta? It's a no-cook, fast prep, make-ahead appetizer that disappears quickly. Make sure you have spreadable breads—crostini, wedges of warmed or baked pita bread, or select from the variety of artisan crackers available at your favorite grocery store.

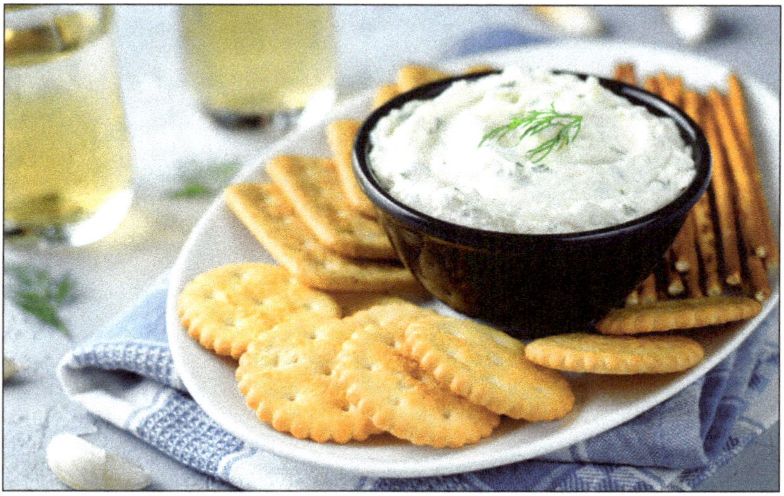

Creamy whipped feta can be added to your charcuterie board, surrounded with cutup veggies and your favorite serving breads. Drizzle with olive oil and/or honey. You can add in capers. One of my favorites is chopped olives—think beyond the standard black olive. Add a kiss of dill or your favorite herb.

If you like nuts, toast some and make available in a small bowl, to add a bit of crunch. Think a full cup of chopped nuts. Have small side dipping bowls that your guests can choose from. The dip is the "main" but all the mini sides add new tastes and flavors.

Add a small cherry or grape tomato medley to your adds. The red, yellow, orange, black, and striped varieties of grapes are fun for your display and flavoring. I love the artesian Bumble Bee brand that brings stripes to your offerings.

Start with a block of feta for this dip, preferably packed in a liquid brine. The wet brine keeps the feta moist and allows for a smooth and creamy dip when blended. Costco carries one that is brined, stored in half inch slices that works and stores well. It's the only American one I use. Fetas that are dry take a lot of work to get to the creamy stage. Avoid. I'm a huge fan of European fetas. The creaminess and moistness is very tasty. Normally, I head to a Middle Eastern grocery store in my area for my "dip star."

makes: 1 cup | **prep time:** 15 minutes | **cooking time:** none

ingredients

8 oz feta (brined) or a Hungarian, French, Bulgarian or Greek
olive oil and/or honey for drizzle
black pepper, coarse
2 T capers, *optional*
herbs—basil, dill, chives, *or your choice*
grape tomatoes, small
olives—Kalamata, black, green
nuts—roasted pecans, almonds, crunched for a fast topping
breads and crackers for dipping, spreading

putting it all together

step 1: Working at room temperature, whip the feta to introduce air. (I whip by hand).

step 2: Add in any herbs you choose. Keep it simple; don't overdo. I also like to add julienned fresh basil to the mix.

step 3: When serving, drizzle olive oil or honey, or sprinkle coarse pepper on top—add other toppings in small bowls. If using capers, mix in with the feta.

With olives, if you use any of the stuffed ones (pimento, garlic), slice some to highlight what's inside and mix with whole ones.

Dip can be stored for a few days in refrigerator. To fluff up again, use a rubber/silicon spatula in a bowl and enjoy a second time.

Gooey Tomato & Cheese Bruschetta

If you are looking for a comfort appetizer, this bruschetta is perfect and simple to put together. In fact, it could be a "dipper" with a bowl of soup or an add to your favorite salad. Meal done!

All you will do is toast slices of baguette, add butter and garlic to one side, then layer with slices of tomato and cheese, and broil for a few minutes until bubbling. Easy peasy? ... so yes!

makes: 20 pieces | **preheat:** oven to broil
prep time: 20 minutes | **cooking time:** 2 minutes or less

ingredients

1 baguette – *you can also use ciabatta or sourdough bread*

½ tsp garlic powder

6 T butter

8 tomatoes, thinly sliced or chopped—*Romas are a good choice here*

Havarti, mozzarella or provolone cheese, shredded

salt and pepper to taste

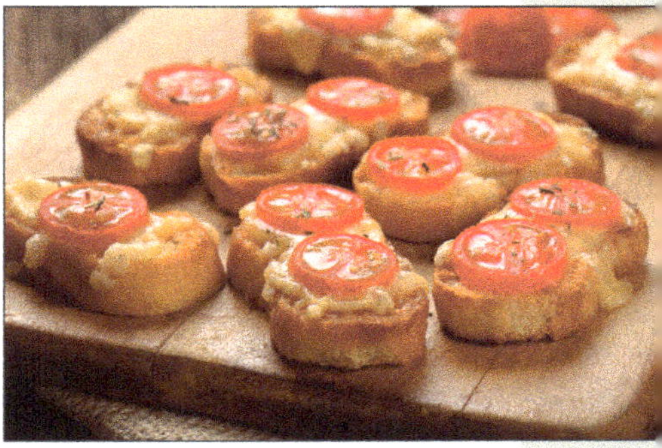

Putting it all together

step 1: Slice baguette ⅜ to ½ inch thick. Thinly slice tomatoes. Slice or shred cheese. Soften butter and mix in garlic.

step 2: Lightly toast baguette slices, both sides.

step 3: Thinly slice tomatoes and slice or shredded cheese. Soften butter and mixed in garlic.

step 4: Broil in the oven for two minutes or less, until the cheese is bubbling. Serve immediately

Peppered Goat Cheese Bruschetta

To me, a bruschetta loaded with flavors is a perfect appetizer. Heck, I've made them a meal. Basil is one of my favorite herbs. For years, I grew my own basil and made my own pesto. When I discovered Costco's Basil Pesto, I said no more. It's close to perfect. My only add is more garlic.

This bruschetta is an ideal add to your appetizer mix as soon as you get your hands on fresh Roma tomatoes. You can always do a substitute with sun dried tomatoes, which delivers a different taste and texture to the bite. The goat cheese has its own tang, and a substitute for it could be one of the Boursin cheeses. Add some fresh cracked pepper on top and serve.

makes: 20 bruschetta | **preheat:** oven to 350°F
prep time: 15 minutes | **cooking time:** 8 minutes

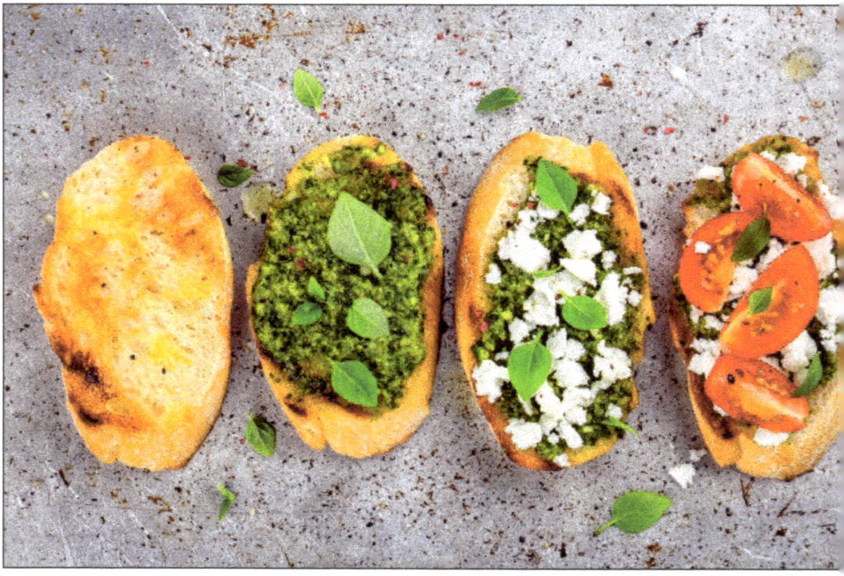

ingredients

1 baguette

1 C basil pesto—*do the cheat and get Costco's*

8 oz goat cheese, soft or crumbled. *Substitute in Boursin if desired.*

3 fresh Roma tomatoes, or sun-dried

2 garlic cloves, minced

½ tsp each salt and pepper

toppings: olive oil, balsamic vinegar, cracked pepper

putting it all together

step 1: Slice baguette to ½- to ⅜-inch thickness.

step 2: Brush both sides of the sliced bread lightly with olive oil. Place on a baking sheet and bake for 6–8 minutes until lightly golden and crispy.

step 3: Dice or slice the tomatoes. Season with minced garlic, salt, and pepper.

step 4: Spread pesto and cheese on toasted sliced baguette pieces. If you are using a soft cheese instead of one you crumble, reverse and spread the cheese first, then the pesto on top.

step 5: Top with diced or sliced tomatoes. Add a final crank of cracked pepper. Serve

Garnish: Drizzle a little olive oil or balsamic vinegar on top with fresh chopped basil or a few basil leaves—use small ones.

Basil, Pine Nuts, Tomato, and Whipped Feta Crostini

Anything crostini is one of my favorites to have as "the appetizer" as the weather warms and I move to my deck to share with friends. Think of these tasty bites as a solo feature, a combo offering of different crostini … or as part of an appetizer spread. This one has a creamy feta base, a mix of cut cherry or grape tomatoes, and, of course, a kiss of basil and pine nuts.

I call for whipped feta here … but a cheat/short cut is to spread softened feta from a block that comes with a brine. Costco carries a good one … or one of the European fetas that is already in a spreadable form as your base. Three of my favorite go-to choices are Bulgarian, French and Hungarian–Bulgarian is the creamiest.

The aroma of basil that is released when I prepare the leaves is one that I love … so much that I have basil plants in my planters close to my front porch.

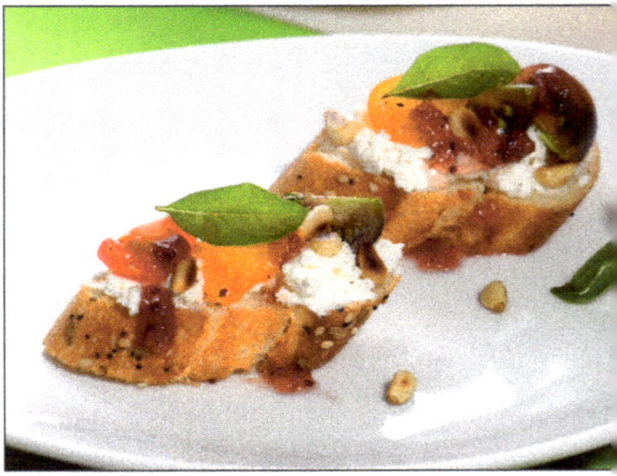

makes: 15 to 25 crostini
preheat: oven to 350°F

ingredients

1 baguette, ¼ to ⅜-inch-thick diagonal baguette slices

for the Whipped Feta

6 oz block of feta

2 oz cream cheese

⅔ C olive oil, divided

2 T lemon juice, fresh

2 T minced shallots (2 shallots)

2 tsp garlic, minced (2 cloves) or ½ tsp garlic powder

2 T red wine vinegar

cherry grape tomatoes, cut in half

basil, fresh

½ C pine nuts, lightly toasted

sea salt and freshly ground black pepper

balsamic vinegar for drizzling

putting it all together

step 1: For toasting/baking your crostini base—stay close to your oven, 5 to 7 minutes max. For pine nuts, a kiss of slightly browning. Also, you can do this in a small frying pan—add 1 tsp melted butter.

This goes fast, so stay put and watch the coloring. Rest to room temperature when done for both.

For the pine nuts and balsamic … quickly toast pine nuts. Have a side small bowl of pine nuts in case someone is nut sensitive. Drizzle a smidge of balsamic vinegar on top of each Crostini … taste and color—just a smidge!

step 2: When working with cheeses, you want them at room temperature to make the whipped feta—both feta and cream cheese.

step 3: For the whipped feta, place the feta and cream cheese in the bowl of a food processor or use a hand mixer. Pulse until mixed. Add ⅓ cup of the olive oil, 2 tablespoons lemon juice, ½ teaspoon salt, and ¼ teaspoon pepper, and process until smooth.

step 4: For the tomatoes, slice or cut in half and marinate an hour ahead, combining the shallots, garlic, and vinegar. Set aside for 5 minutes. Whisk in the remaining olive oil, 1 teaspoon salt, and pepper. Gently stir in cut tomatoes and set aside for 10 minutes. Stir in any basil if you choose to julienne several leaves. Taste.

step 5: To assemble the crostini, spread each slice of bread with a generous amount of whipped feta. Tomatoes. Drizzle with balsamic, and a leaf or two of basil. I put the pine nuts in a small bowl in case someone has a nut allergy.

Naan Crisps with a Kick

Skip the store package chips … make your own.

You can easily bake naan bread into crispy, crunchy looks like "pita chips." Because naan is thicker and softer, your chip with have plenty of flavor and will hold up well when it's dipped or your dip is spooned on. I love the minis—you can either bake them flat or add some flair and push them into a mini muffin tin to add a scooping curve to your crisps.

Naan is thicker and softer than pita. I thank my foodie friend, Juliana, for introducing me to Cran-Peño pepper jelly—it is perfect to add a smidge of kick—and the idea of using the mini muffin pan to create the curves on the crisps. It's her photo we used here. Also consider adding the Whipped Feta or even a Greek Tzatziki. Heck, why not have a few dip options?

makes: 30–40 crisps | **preheat:** oven to 375°F
prep time: less than 10 minutes | **cooking time:** 10-13 minutes

ingredients

1½ lbs (around 20 oz) naan – *use the minis or large bread cut into wedges—get the Stonefire at Costco. Remember to refrigerate until you use.*

½ C olive oil

1 tsp garlic powder

½ C Parmesan, grated

¾ tsp sea salt

¾ tsp pepper

½ tsp paprika

Dipping sauces: Cran-Peño Jalapeño Preserves, **Greek Tzatziki** (recipe follows), **Whipped Feta** page 35.

putting it all together

step 1: With a knife or pizza cutter, cut the naan into bite-sized wedges.

step 2: Whisk olive oil, garlic salt, pepper, and paprika together and brush naan generously.

step 3: Single layer the wedges on a baking sheet or use a mini muffin tin and push in your pieces. Bake for 10-15 minutes, or until lightly golden.

step 4: Cool on baking sheet or in muffin tin completely before using or storing for use later. The cooling process adds to the crispness.

step 5: On to a platter or into a festive bowl with the offer of a few sauces. I like the Cran-Peño or think about a **Greek Tzatziki** (recipe follows) or the **Whipped Feta** on page 35

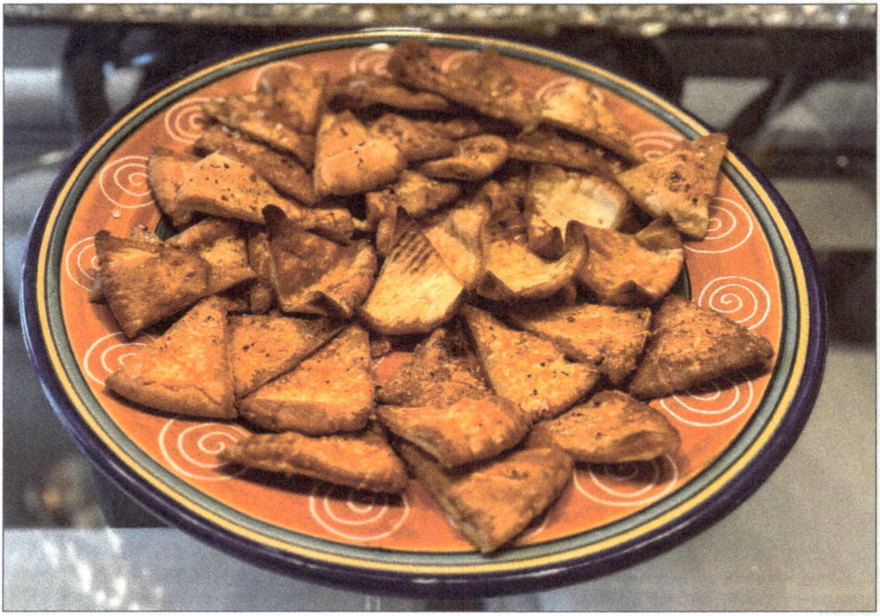

Greek Tzatziki

Don't make this sauce at the last minute … you want to mix all ingredients together for an overnight date in your refrigerator. This one needs blending time.

yield: 2 cups

ingredients

½ of a large seedless cucumber — *don't peel*

1½ C plain full-fat Greek yogurt

2 large garlic cloves, minced

2 T extra virgin olive oil

1 T white vinegar

½ tsp sea salt

1 T fresh dill, minced — *you will add this to the sauce just before serving*

putting it all together

step 1: Grate the cucumber and drain through a fine mesh sieve to press out more of the liquid.

step 2: Combine the yogurt, garlic, oil, vinegar, and salt in a bowl. Cover and refrigerate overnight.

step 3: Add the grated cucumber and fresh dill to the yogurt mixture and stir to combine. Dill can sometimes overwhelm, so I add it just before serving. Back to the refrigerator for a short chill. Serve with naan crisps for dipping.

The tzatziki can last for about 3-4 days.

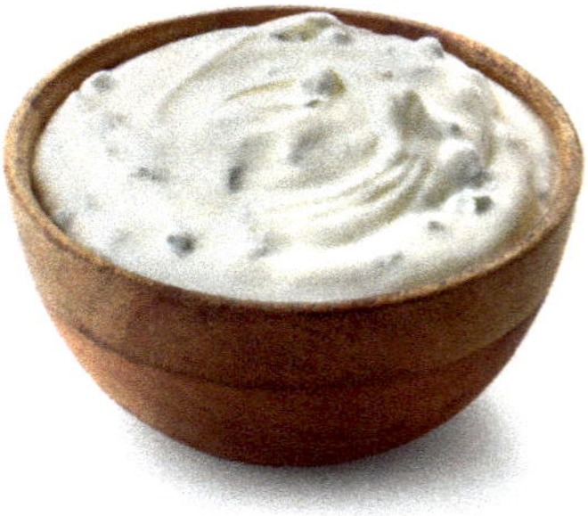

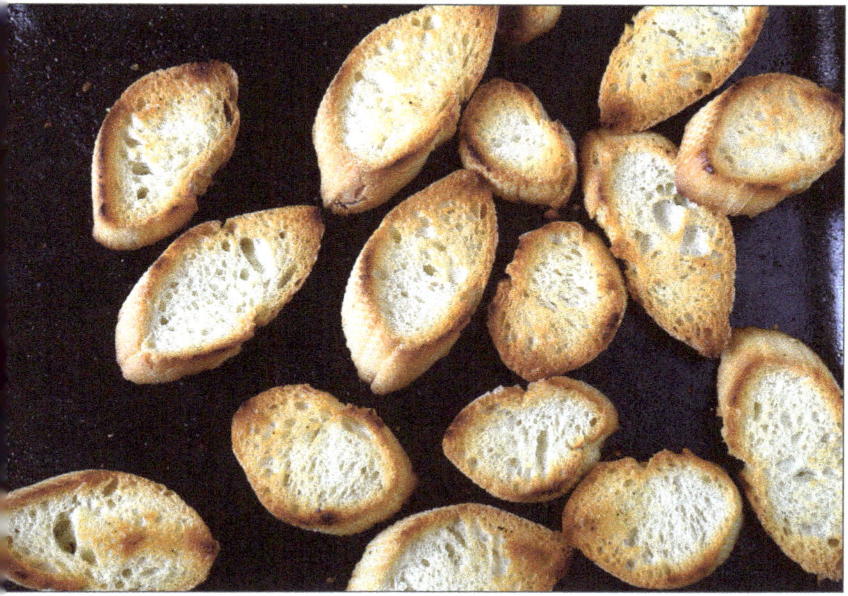

Crostini

Bread is a constant in the appetizer mix. My favorite is a crostini —it's the perfect base to showcase your favorite dip or creamy spread. Here's the bonus: leftovers can be crunched into salads for croutons and added to top of your favorite soup. Once you start making your own ... you will not go back to the prepackaged store-bought variety. So boring.

Crostini means "little toasts" or "little crusts" in Italian. They are usually smaller, round, or created from a baguette. Sliced. Oiled. Baked. Perfect for finger food and are eater friendly. When I'm making a batch and a friend is visiting, she typically hit my drawer with sandwich zippered storage bags ... "I'll just take a few to nibble on the drive home ..."Why not!

You may also come across another Italian word: bruschetta. The bread is a little thicker and almost soaked in olive oil and garlic. When it's in the bruschetta realm—one or two per guests. Crostini? At least three!

makes: 20–25 crostini

preheat: oven to 375°F | **prep time:** 15 minutes

cook time: 8-10 minutes or until toasted and golden brown

ingredients

1 baguette

½ C olive oil

1 tsp garlic powder

Sea salt to taste

putting it all together

step 1: Use a serrated knife to cut the bread into ¼-inch thick slices—thick enough to hold all the toppings but thin enough to easily bite into once toasted.

step 2: Lay the slices on a lined sheet pan (no parchment) and use a pastry brush to generously coat each piece with olive oil-garlic mix—just brush one side, it will soak through. Include the sides of the bread.

step 3: Sprinkle each slice with sea salt.

step 4: Bake. I store crostini in an airtight container for up to three days.

Toasty Caprese Crostini

Transform the classic caprese into bite-sized finger food by making Toasty Caprese Crostini. Of course, you can add other foodie elements, but I would keep this fairly simple. I like the sliced black olives for color contrast, texture, and added taste. Toast slices of baguette or sourdough, layer with slices of tomato, and broil for a few minutes with fresh mozzarella until bubbling.

Rarely are crostinis a solo appetizer act. Think a trio of bite size delights, giving your guests an "I want them all" to the "just one" option. I love to mix colors, textures, and varieties when I do this. Cheese and bread are here ... add one of the veggie appetizers and one of the seafood or meat choices.

This is ideal for the early afternoon friends who have skipped lunch or the later gang who have the "hungry" look in their eyes!

makes: 20 to 25 crostini | **preheat:** oven to broil
prep time: 20 minutes | **cooking time:** 2 minutes

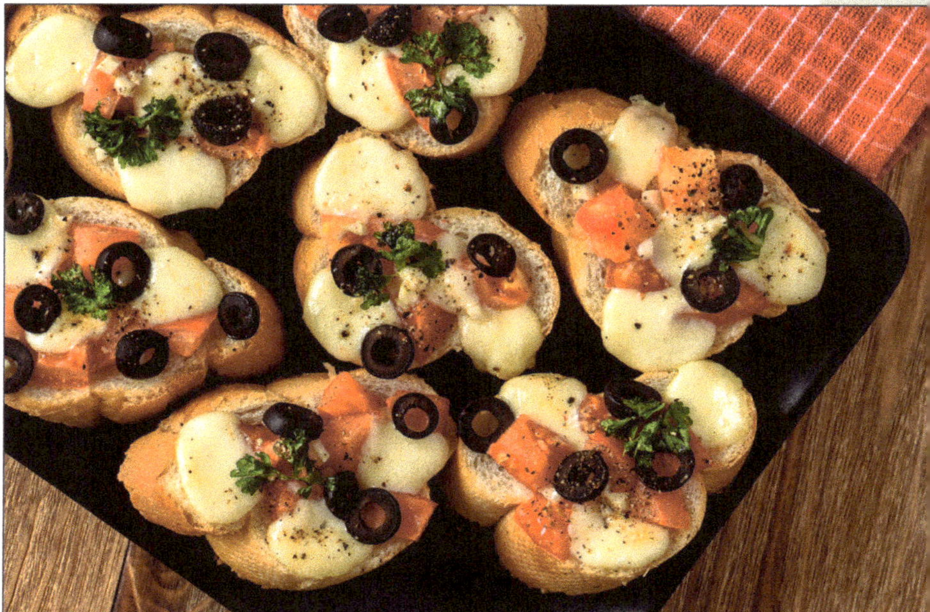

ingredients

1 baguette—*you can also use ciabatta or sourdough bread*

½ tsp garlic powder

6 T butter

8 tomatoes, thinly sliced or chopped—*Romas are a good choice here*

½ can black olives, sliced

mozzarella or provolone cheese, shredded

salt and pepper to taste

basil, chopped

putting it all together

step 1: Slice baguette ⅜ to ½ inch thick.

step 2: Slice olives and tomatoes. Soften butter and stir in garlic.

step 3: Lightly toast slices, both sides.

step 4: Spread a thin layer of garlic-herb butter on one side. Top with thinly sliced tomatoes (two per baguette slice) and top generously with shredded mozzarella or provolone. Add olives.

step 5: Broil in the oven for two minutes or until the cheese is bubbling. Garnish with fresh basil, salt, and pepper.

The 10-Minute Rule when using fresh garlic in cooking:
When you crush, chop, or mince fresh garlic, let it rest at room temperature for about 10 minutes before cooking. Magic happens. The waiting period allows enzymes to convert garlic compounds into allicin, which is responsible for the ingredient's distinct flavor and health benefits.

Sweet Heat Cranberry and Honey Puff Pastry Baked Brie

Anything Brie ranks high in my foodie offerings when it is displayed. It spreads easily at room temps and when warmed for me, moves into my divine arena. Adding puff pastry into the mix, a filling or a topping all works.

My friend, Juliana, is like me—the two of us can create an entire meal around appetizers. One of her "go-to's" is a Sweet Heat Cranberry & Honey Puff Pastry Baked Brie and now it is one of mine. And I think this will be one of yours.

A small Brie is 3 to 4 inches in diameter and consists of 3 to 4 ounces of cheese. Medium is 5-7 inches and contains 8-12 ounces of cheese. Most likely, you will be using the medium size. Of course, there are larger ones. If you use one, increase your proportions and double the puff pastry. This is when I eyeball it.

serves: 2 to 4, small Brie | medium Brie 4 to 8
preheat: oven to 350°F | **prep time:** 10 minutes
cooking time: 10-14 minutes until golden and cheese oozes

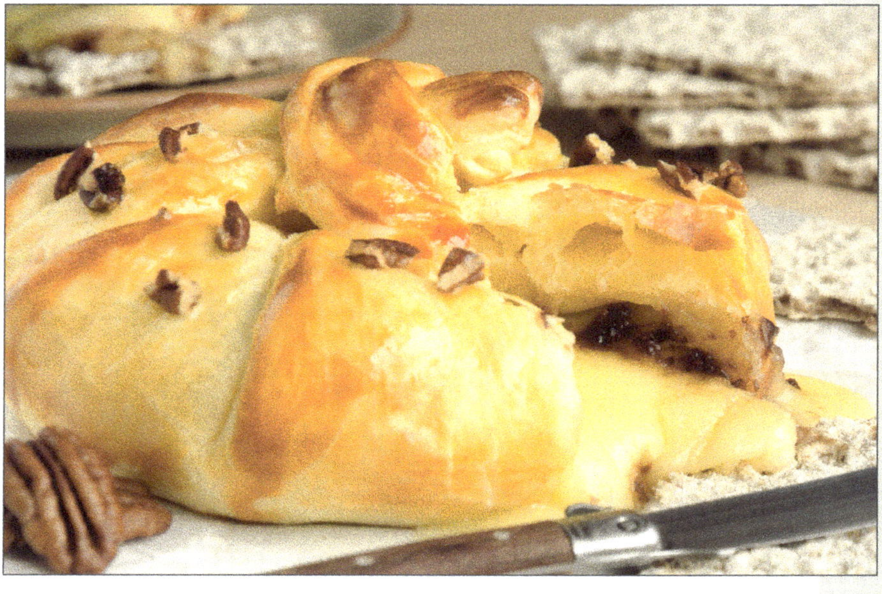

ingredients

1 Brie, medium size

puff pastry sheets frozen—*made with butter only. One sheet is more than adequate for a small Brie, two for medium or large Brie.*

½ – ¾ C cranberries, fresh or frozen

¼ C walnuts or pecans

¼ C pickled onions or ¼ C green onions, chopped

2 – 3 T Sweet Heat or Cran-Peño Jelly
(Amazon has a huge selection)

¼ C sun-dried tomatoes, cut into small pieces

1 egg

Note: For a sweeter flavor, add a dollop of honey or fig jam

putting it all together

Bries come with a white rind around. It is edible, but many prefer it removed or at least removed from most of the Brie or at least the top layer. When I do this, I use dental floss.

step 1: The night before you are planning on making the Brie, take the puff pastry out of freezer and defrost it in the fridge.

step 2: Remove the defrosted puff pastry and let rest for at least 10 minutes to bring to room temperature. Remove the top layer of the rind. Bring the pastry to room temp prior to manipulating it to cover the Brie.

step 3: Sprinkle a small amount of flour on a SilPat baking mat or your prep surface—mine is a granite counter. If two pieces of pastry are used for a larger round of Brie, then these will have to be gently pressed together.

step 4: Next spread 2-3 T of Sweet Heat or Cran-Peño on top of the Brie with mixture of onions, tomatoes, cranberries, and nuts. If a sweeter flavor is desired, add a dollop of honey or fig jam.

step 5: Place your Brie with its toppings in the center of the puff pastry. Leave a small opening in the puff pastry on the top for a vent as you cover the rest of the pastry around the Brie.

step 6: Place your encased Brie on a pan lined with parchment paper, and brush with one egg mixed with a fork and spread on top of pastry top and sides. Bake for 10-14 minutes until golden brown and cheese is beginning to ooze out over the vented top.

Serve with favorite crackers, sliced baguettes, pita chips, naan, or crostini.

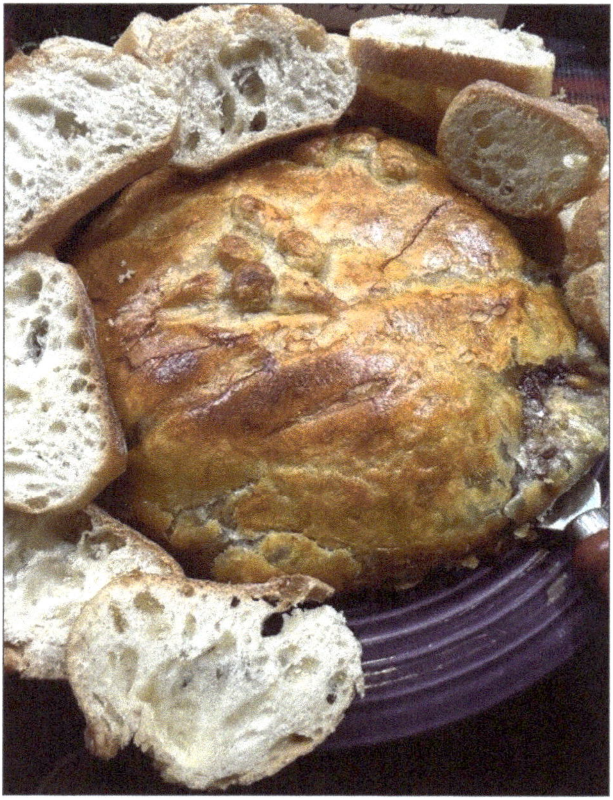

Of all the things I loved
over my decades of living,
partnerships, and unions …
food has been the longest relationship!

— Judith Briles

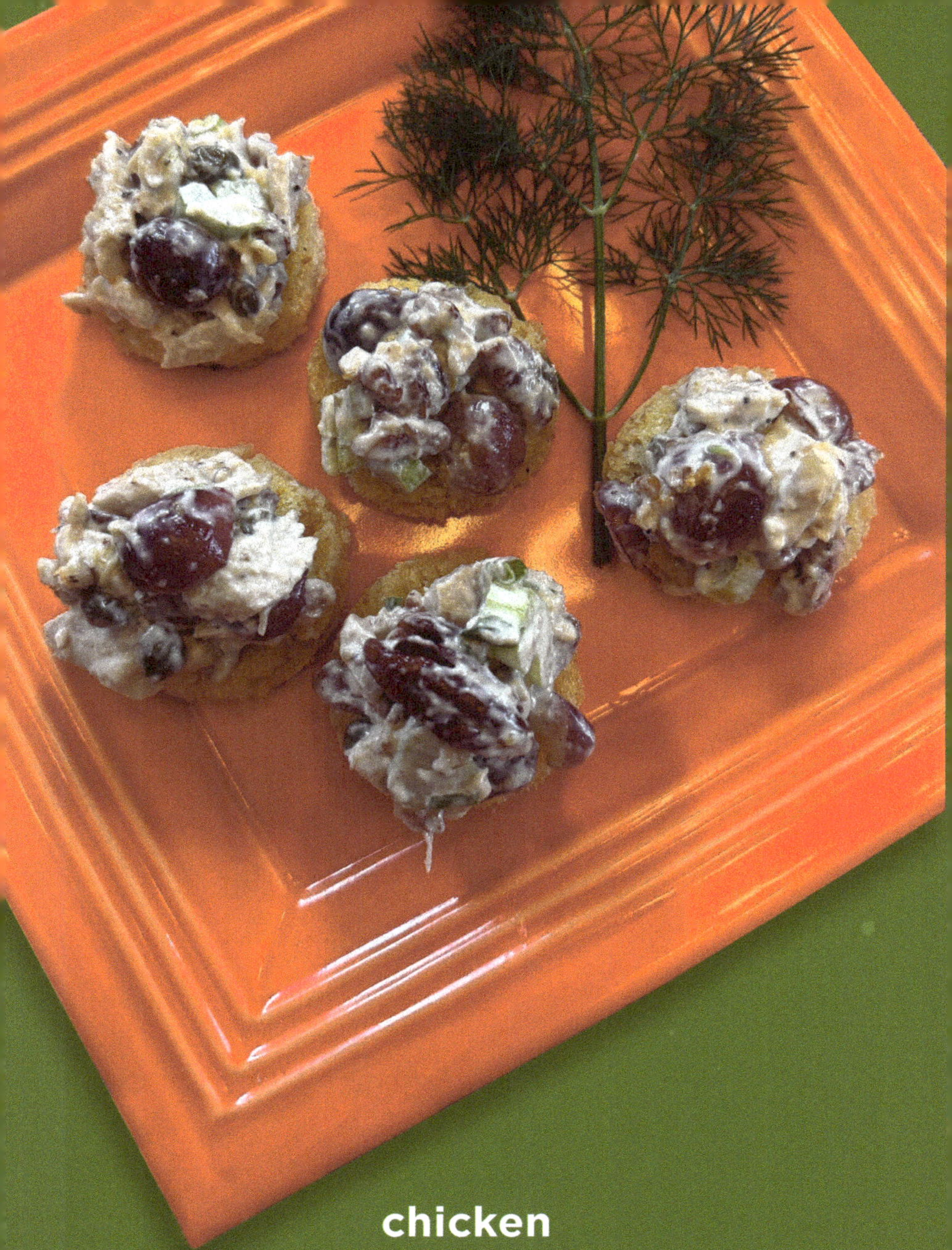

chicken

Chicken Salad Sliders

If you are a slider fan, my Chicken Salad Sliders always remind me of my love of Hawaii. It's the pineapple, the crunch of the macadamia nuts, and the Hawaiian butter rolls that reinforce it. An added surprise is the banana peppers that give each bite a smidge of savory punch to the mix. For me, it's like adding a tad of sunshine to what my guests enjoy. Although I prefer the thigh to the breast, I suggest you do a combo—mixing both into your spread. You can cook your own chicken, get a rotisserie one (I get one from Costco) and pull it apart. Or you can even use canned chicken—that leaves you with a white breast only option.

If you are thinking of a lunchtime, afternoon gathering, or early evening during the summer months, do an appetizer trio combo: include the Watermelon, Feta, and Basil Bites and the Hawaiian Bruschetta. Perfect.

makes: 8 to 16 Sliders | **prep time:** 30 minutes

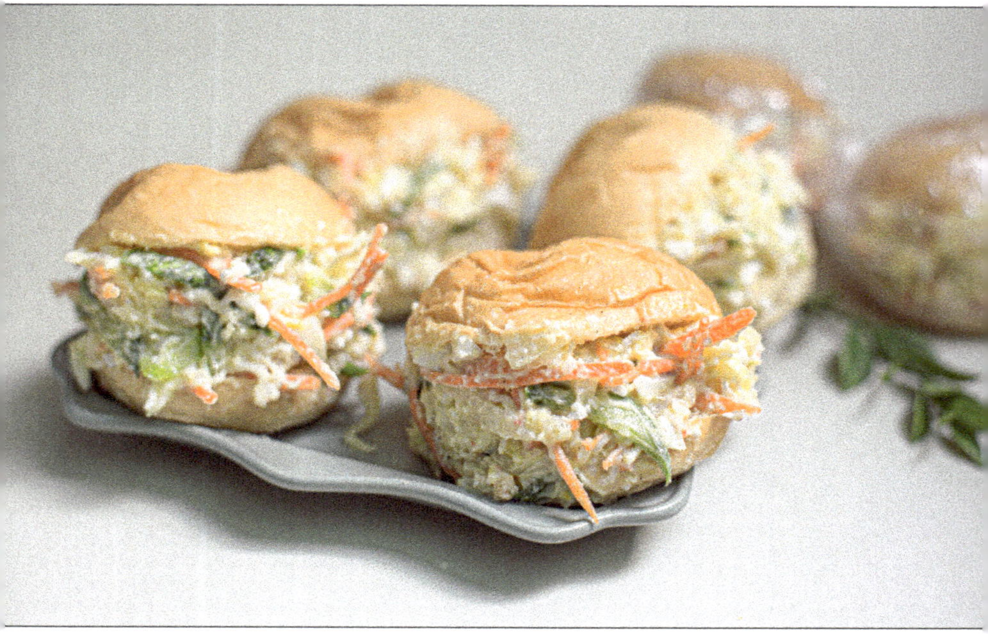

ingredients

2 C chicken, thigh and breast, cooked and chopped

1 C pineapple, crushed and drained

½ C celery, chopped

½ C carrots, shredded

1 C grapes, seedless, red or green

½ C macadamia nuts, chopped

½ C banana peppers, pickled rings

½ to 1 C mayonnaise

2 T parsley, chopped

1 tsp celery salt

¼ tsp salt

½ tsp black pepper

8 to 16 King's Hawaiian dinner rolls

putting it all together

step 1: Make salad filling by combining all ingredients except the dinner rolls. Refrigerate 1 hour.

step 2: Slice the rolls in half, separating the tops from the bottoms. Lightly toast the insides for an added layer of filling support and a layer of crunch for your guests.

step 3: Spoon in a generous layer of filling. Before adding top of the roll, include a sweetish pepper surprise—slip in a banana pepper ring (or two).

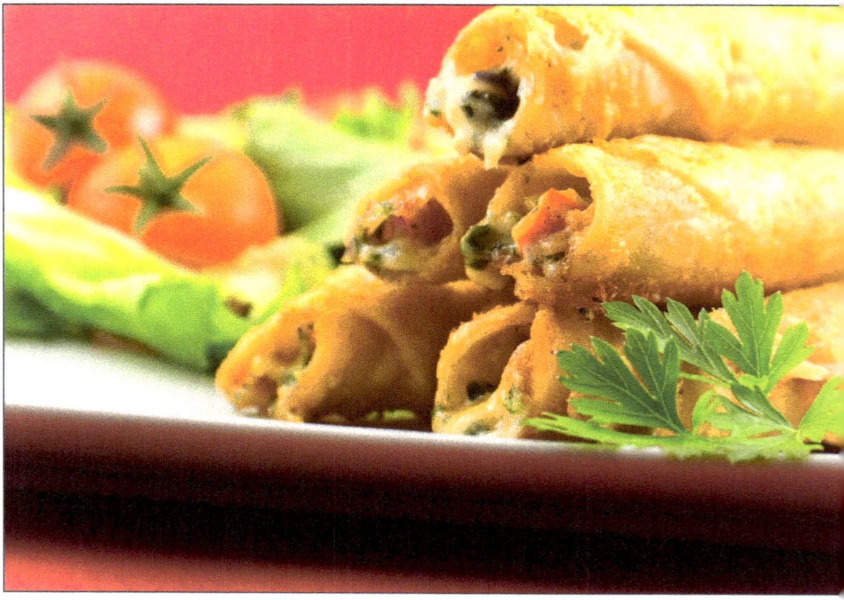

Chicken Veggie Taquitos … Olé!

Since my first bite, I have always liked taquitos. Most are beef or chicken. Sometimes with veggies added—a Mexican type of spring roll. Can be served with a tortilla, to fry quickly, or baked. Make them more bite size by cutting them in half lengthwise before baking. Either way, your guests will welcome them, and your serving will disappear.

Plan on 3 to 4 bite-sized taquitos per person—that's 1 to 2 whole taquitos. I typically cut them in half. This recipe is to make the taquito from scratch. There's aways the cheat—you can buy them frozen from the grocery store and just add the guacamole.

makes: 20 Taquito halves | **preheat:** oven to 425°F

prep time: 15-20 minutes | **stove top cooking time:** 15 minutes

ingredients

15 corn tortillas

vegetable or avocado oil

1 yellow onion, finely chopped

1 each red and yellow bell pepper, finely chopped

½ package of taco seasoning

2 T butter or vegetable oil

½ C chicken broth

½ C salsa, green or red - thick

2 chicken breasts or 4 thighs, boneless and skinless

3 oz cream cheese

1–2 C cheddar cheese, grated

Garnishes: avocados to make guacamole, cilantro, green onions. sour cream, salsa

putting it all together

step 1: Heat the oil in a large skillet. Add the onions and peppers and sauté until tender. Add the chicken and taco seasoning, salsa, and broth.

Cover, reduce the heat, and simmer for 10 minutes. Remove the chicken and shred it; then return to the skillet, adding in cream cheese and half of the cheddar cheese until the two are melted. Remove from heat and allow it to cool.

step 2: Fill the flat tortilla, add cheddar and a few green onions, and roll tightly.

step 3: On a baking sheet, either sprayed with a non-aerosol oil or lined with parchment paper, lay your taquitos out. You will bake for 10-14 minutes … turn halfway through.

Serve with sour cream, salsa, green onions, cilantro, and/or guacamole for dipping.

Guacamole

makes: 1–1½ cups depending on size of avocados

2 avocados, ripe and smashed

1 tomato, chopped

½ lime, juiced

2 T salsa of your choice, approximately

salt to taste

green onion

step 1: Mash avocado—*I usually do with a fork*—it does not have to be smooth. I like a few chunks.

step 2: Add tomato and diced green onion to mashed avocado. Blend.

step 3: Add 2 tablespoons of salsa. Gently blend and taste. *Does it need salt?* Add a few shakes from your salt shaker and taste again. *More?* Repeat.

step 4: Squeeze one-half lime on top just before serving.

Note: I make guacamole no more than 30 minutes before serving. So it is fresh and not threatening to brown.

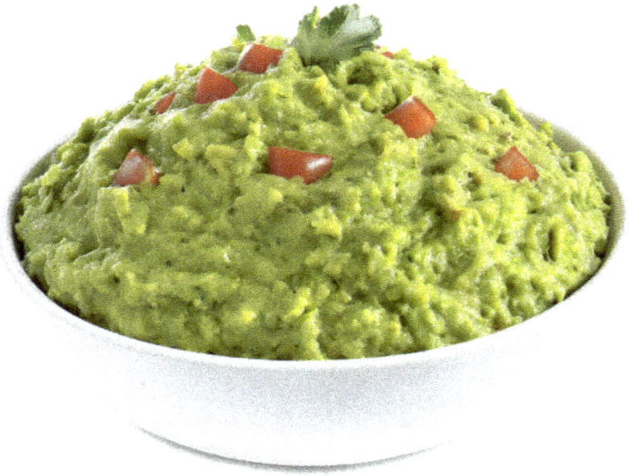

Wicked and Wimpy Chicken Wings

Chicken wings are quickly devoured at gatherings. Often fried—take a pass and bake them instead. You can make your sauce on the wicked side or just a simple taste for those of us who want to wimp out. If you are really wimpy, mosey over to your grocery store and create your own Wing Board Feast with lots of options to dip into.

Do not just have the Wicked sauce version. Those of us who are on the Wimpy side don't want a firehose of heat coming at us. For me, I'm a Bleu Cheese or Sweet & Sour type of gal. Make your own … or check out the variety of options at your favorite grocery store.

makes: 20 to 24 wings | **preheat:** oven to 450°F
(you will drop temperature to 375°F for second stage of cooking)
prep time: 30 minutes | **cooking time:** 22 minutes

ingredients

20 to 24 chicken wings … drums and flats

2 T garlic powder

2 T extra virgin olive oil

½ tsp smoked paprika

2 large garlic cloves, finely grated

kosher salt

2 T unsalted butter

lime wedges, for serving

Nonstick cooking spray, for the baking sheets

2 shallots, diced

1 C ketchup

1 lime, juiced

1 tsp ginger

1 tsp mustard, poupon or yellow

5 shakes hot sauce—*I use Cholula*

putting it all together

step 1: Wings cook fast in the oven. 450°F for 10 minutes to allow the skin to crisp up. Reduce oven to 350°F for another 8-12 minutes to finish cooking.

step 2: In a large bowl, combine and coat the chicken with the garlic powder, olive oil, smoked paprika, grated garlic, and a generous pinch of salt.

step 3: Line two baking sheets with parchment paper and spray the parchment with nonstick spray. Arrange the chicken wings in a single layer with space between each. You want space between the wings for browning.

step 4: In a small pan, heat the olive oil, then add the shallots and garlic to simmer for 3-4 minutes. Stir in the ketchup and lightly cook for 2 minutes to intensify the taste. Whisk in the ginger, mustard, hot sauce, and lime juice.

step 5: Bake for 10 minutes. Lower the heat to 375°F and bake until cooked through, 8-12 minutes more. After cooking, separate the wings you want for your Wicked sauce choice, and put aside some for those who prefer the Less Wicked or Wimpy sauce option. Add all the sauces on next page or sub in another—it's your choice.

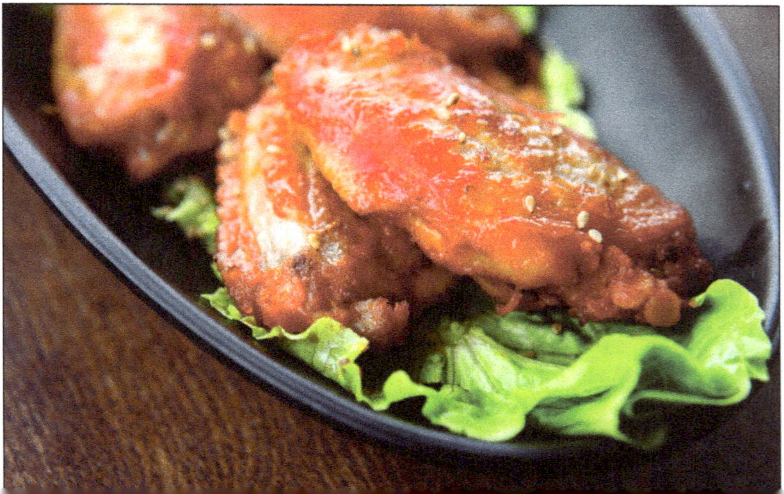

Wicked Sauce

makes: 1½ cups

1 C mayonnaise

1 T buttermilk

3 T onions, minced or 2 tsp onion powder

1 tsp cracked pepper

1 tsp garlic powder

1 T Dijon mustard, smooth or coarse

1-2 T hot sauce

1 tsp ginger

1 tsp paprika

putting it all together

Mix all of the ingredients above. Add hot sauce to taste—more means MORE heat. *Suggestion … start with just a little … let it rest, then add more if desired.* Heat the sauce. Toss the cooked chicken to coat and serve.

Less Wicked Sauce

makes: ¾ cup

1 T extra virgin olive oil

2 medium shallots, minced

2 large garlic cloves, finely grated

½ C ketchup

1 T fresh ginger, grated

1 T Dijon mustard

1 T sweet chili sauce

1 tsp hot sauce

2 limes, juiced

kosher salt to taste

putting it all together

Mix all together and do the same process as above. Make sure you label them for your guests.

Wimpy: Sweet & Sour Ranch Sauce

makes: 1½ cups

1 C (8 oz) sour cream

¼ C buttermilk

¼ C mayonnaise

2 T chopped fresh dill

2 T honey

2 T apple cider vinegar

2 tsp garlic powder

2 tsp onion powder

2 tsp Worcestershire sauce

putting it all together

For the Wimpy side, combine all the Wimpy ingredients. Cook the wings and serve with the dressing. Provide lime wedges on the side.

Cashew Chicken Curry Crostini

If you like a little salty, sweet, chewy, and a bit of crunch, here's a quick and easy appetizer to put together and please your guests. Chicken with a kiss of curry and a nibble of cashew nuts and a smidge of apricot is a great add to your finger food offerings. It's fast and easy when you have leftover roasted chicken or pick one up at your local grocery store.

Bonus ... it's great as a salad for lunch with your favorite lettuce choice!

makes: 20 to 25 crostini | **preheat:** oven to 375°F for crostini
prep time: for topping 15 minutes | **cook time:** 8-10 minutes

ingredients

baguette, sliced ¼ to ⅜ inch thick

2 to 3 C chicken, cooked thigh and breast, chopped or shredded

½ C celery, finely chopped

⅓ C red onion, finely chopped

3 T apricot preserves

½ to 1 C mayonnaise or a combo of 1 C Greek plain yogurt and ½ C mayonnaise

1½ T white wine vinegar

½ C cashews, roasted and chopped

1 T curry powder

1 tsp celery salt

½ tsp black pepper

cilantro, chopped

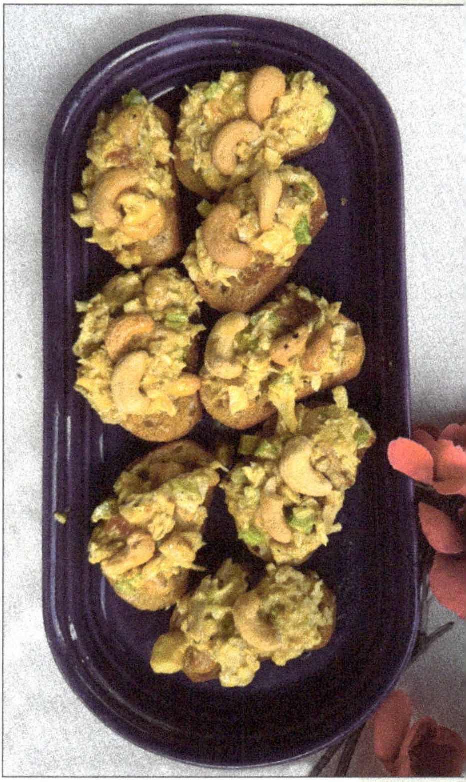

putting it all together

step 1: Make crostini with baguette slices. Brush both sides with olive oil, sprinkle with a pinch of garlic salt and pepper. Bake at 375°F for 5 minutes per side.

step 2: Whisk the curry powder, yogurt, mayonnaise, one tablespoon of apple cider vinegar, apricot preserves, and salt. Taste. Add more curry if desired.

step 3: Blend in the shredded chicken.

Refrigerate until ready to serve. Add a generous teaspoon of the Cashew Chicken Curry on top of each crostini.

To serve: Include a small bowl of chopped cilantro by your platter for guests to add if they choose.

eggs

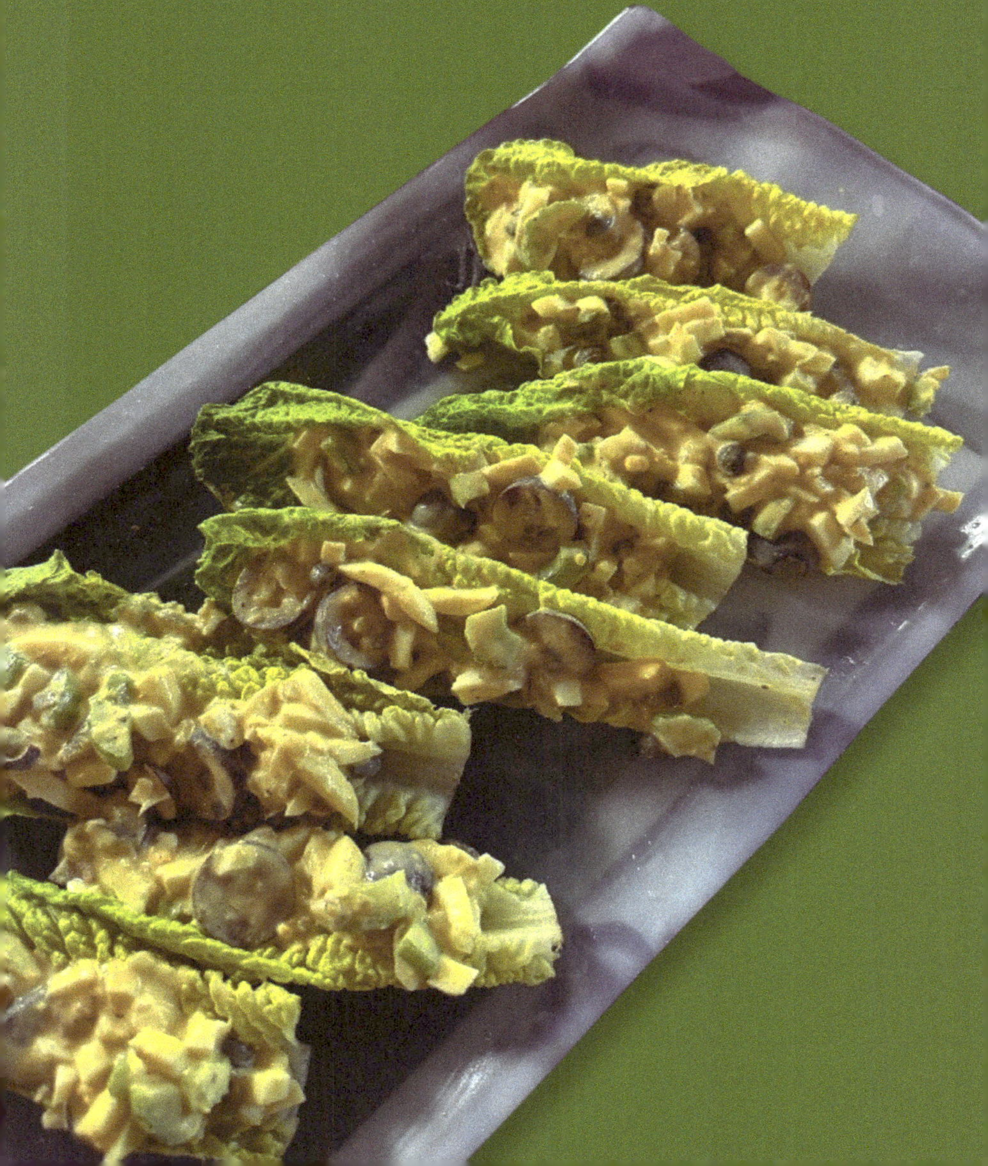

Deviled Eggs … Capers, Curry, or Spice

The perfect deviled egg isn't about complicated techniques or fancy ingredients. No, it's about getting the basics right and then adding one or two ingredients to make them interesting and perk them up. Deviled egg halves disappear fast at any get-together.

For me, my basic deviled egg always includes mayonnaise, Dijon mustard, salt, and pepper. Then I add capers and some chives. I could do a switch and add curry powder for a different version. Or I could bypass the capers and chives and go the spicy route, subbing in a dab of hot sauce and red chili flakes or a bit of jalapeño. I add pieces of cooked bacon on top when I make a tray of mixed deviled eggs—something for everyone!

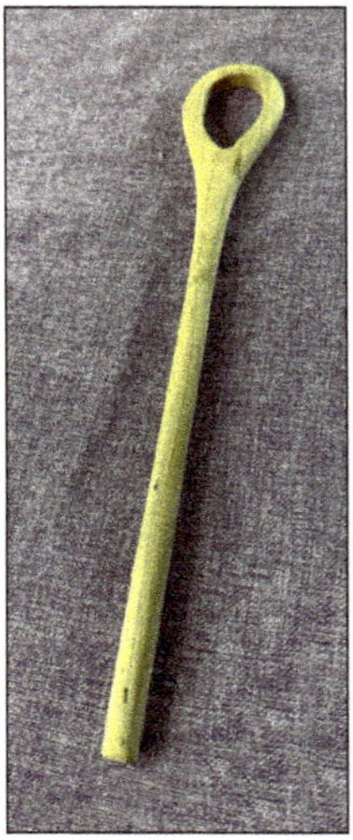

Whatever you choose, you will blend in with the BASIC. Some pipe it into the egg cavities. I'm not for cleaning bags, so a zippered storage bag with a corner cut out to squeeze the mixture through works fine. In reality, I'm from the old school and teaspoon it. It's your choice.

At higher altitudes, water's boiling point is lower—meaning it takes longer to cook an egg.

At sea level, a hard boil takes 10–12 minutes; higher levels should add another minute for every 1,000 feet of altitude. I live at 6,200 feet, so I boil for 16 to 18 minutes.

Big Tip *for easy peeling of eggs … do not use "new" eggs. I buy mine at least one week before I need them and keep in the refrigerator. When hard-boiling, boil water FIRST and then gently transfer raw eggs into the boiling water. I have a special wooden spoon with a rimmed hole to do this. It recently celebrated 50 years of living in my kitchen. And … never put wood in your dishwasher.*

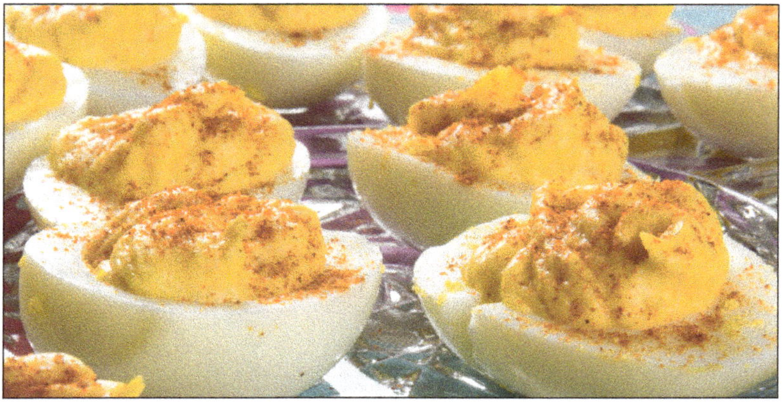

The Basic Egg

makes: 24 egg halves

prep time: 20 minutes | **cooking time:** 13 minutes

ingredients

12 large eggs, hard-boiled

¾ C mayonnaise

1 T Dijon mustard

salt and freshly ground black pepper to taste

paprika sprinkled on top of filled egg

Refrigerate until ready to serve.

Capers and Chives—*my go-to*

additional prep time: 30 minutes

ingredients

3 T of capers

3 T chives, divided—*I use my kitchen scissors to quickly cut. Keep about 1T for sprinkling on top.*

paprika, for sprinkling

Add to your BASIC and fill your egg halves. Top with more chives and a sprinkle of paprika.

Curry—*be different*

additional prep time: 20 minutes

ingredients

1½ tsp curry powder

1–2 T mango chutney—*I use Major Grey's.*

Add to your BASIC and fill your egg halves. Top with a dab of the chutney on top.

Spicy—*add an olé to your eggs*

additional prep time: 30 minutes

ingredients

1 T Cholula or sriracha sauce—*more if you want to increase the heat*

1 T jalapeño, seeded and slivered

1-2 T fresh chives, minced

Add to your BASIC and fill your egg halves. Top with one or two small pieces of jalapeño and/or more chives.

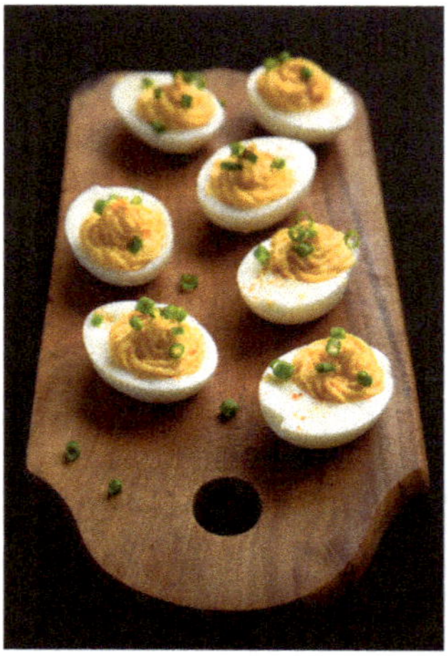

Capers and Chives

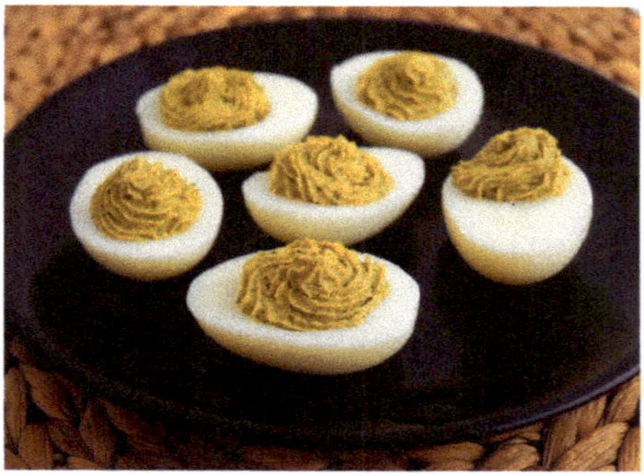

Curry eggs

putting it all together

step 1: Fill a saucepan with enough water to cover eggs by an inch and bring to a full boil. Carefully lower eggs into boiling water. Let eggs boil uncovered for about 30 seconds. Reduce the heat to low and cover. Simmer for 12 minutes. Transfer boiled eggs to a bowl of cold or ice water.

step 2: When cool enough to handle, gently break the shell apart and peel. I start the crack at the narrow end of the egg. If possible, refrigerate eggs overnight, which makes them easier to cut.

step 3: Once cool, cut in half lengthwise with a very sharp knife. Carefully spoon yolks out into a small bowl and arrange whites on a serving platter.

step 4: In a medium bowl, mash yolks into a paste with the back of a fork. Add mayonnaise, mustard; whisk until smooth. Season to taste with salt and freshly ground black pepper. Spoon or pipe filling into egg white halves.

Cover and refrigerate eggs for 2 hours or more, up to 1 day. Once chilled, sprinkle with what you choose to accent—more chives, paprika, cilantro. Serve.

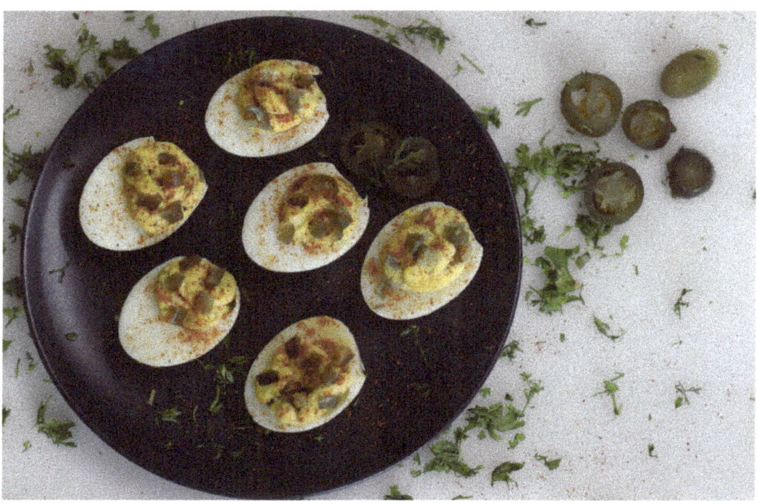

Spicy eggs

Egg Salad Boats

Think of my Egg Salad Boats as a perfect appetizer or mini salad bites. I served them the first time with diced chicken as the main ingredient at a party of about 20 people at a Friday neighborhood gathering. They were scooped up quickly and one of my guests asked if I had extras in my other refrigerator. "Why?" I asked.

"I have a party to go to tonight and need to bring something. If you have any extras, I'll buy them from you," was her response.

"If I did, how many would you need?"

Ten was her answer. "I will make them for you. I have the leaves and filling. It will take me less than 10 minutes to put it altogether for you … and it will be a gift from me to you." And so, I did.

As I gathered ideas for this book, my thoughts were—Why not take the popular Chicken Salad Boats and substitute in my egg salad concoction? I had another Friday gathering at the end of the week and decided I would appeal to all those who love deviled eggs. It worked. I promise, there will be no leftovers.

makes: 20 boats

prep time: 20 minutes | **cooking time:** 20 minutes

ingredients

baby Romaine lettuce—*endive also works*

2 C chopped hard-boiled eggs

1 C mayonnaise

3 T capers

½ C relish, sweet or dill

½ C olives, sliced—*your choice of type*

1 T dill or 1 T curry powder … *or split the mayo, eggs, capers, relish, and do a half and half*

salt and pepper to taste

paprika to sprinkle on top

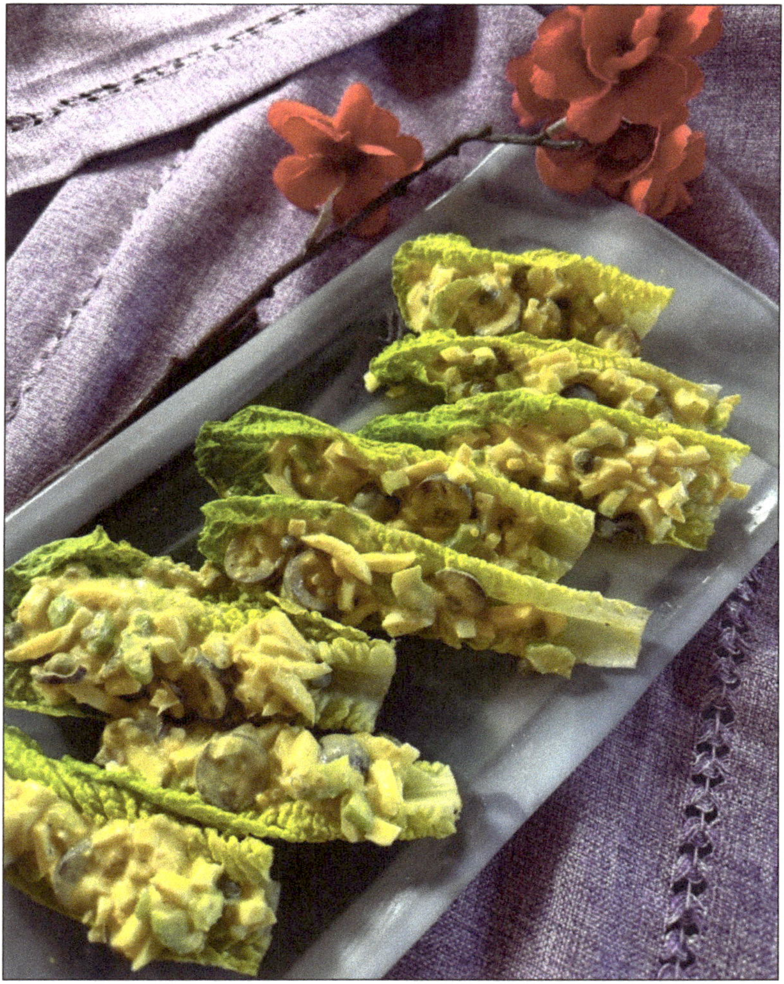

putting it all together

step 1: Boil the eggs, cool, and peel as in **The Basic Egg** on page 67.

step 2: Dice them up. Mix all other ingredients.

step 3: Scoop onto leaves. Sprinkle with a kiss of paprika. I usually do all this a few hours before I plan on serving, as a make-ahead. Refrigerate until serving.

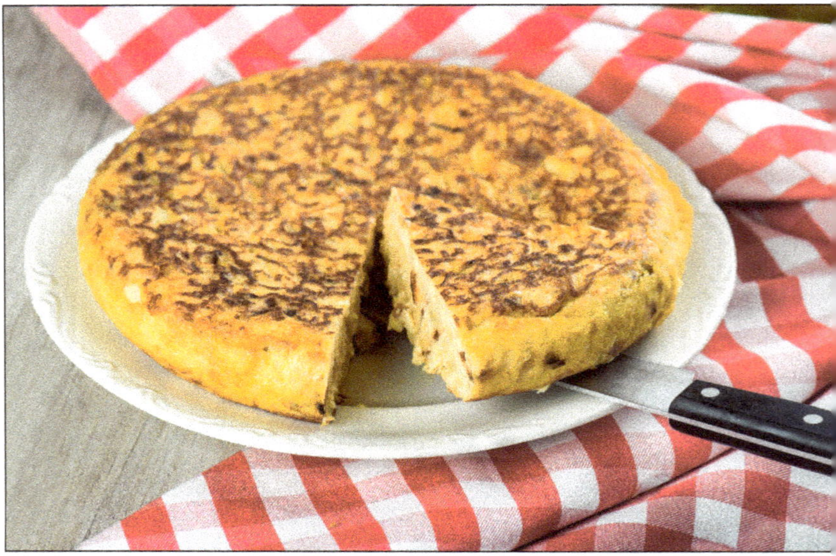

Potato Spanish Omelet

The Spanish omelet is called tortilla de patatas. Think of it as a Spanish tortilla, potato omelet, even a frittata. Many think of it as Spain's national dish.

My Scottish secretary introduced me to a variation of this. When visiting Barcelona, it was a routine tapa at the local bars. Needless to say, it's one of my favorites. This is my variation. And it does take time to put all together.

Use a frying pan with an 8 to 9 inch diameter … or, if you use a larger one … be prepared to just shape your finished omelet with your hands. It's a very "casual" dish … perfect nibbling food while schmoozing with friends at the end of the day with a preferred beverage. Mine is peach iced tea. Yours … Sangria, vino … what?

makes: 8 slices

prep time: 25 minutes | **cooking time:** 45-60 minutes, on stovetop

ingredients

4–5 large Yukon Gold potatoes peeled and sliced ⅛ inch thick

1 large onion, thinly sliced

6 large pimiento-stuffed olives, thinly sliced or chopped

1 red pepper, cut & chopped

2 garlic cloves, chopped—
of course, garlic lovers can go for more!

5 large eggs

1 C olive oil

coarse salt and pepper, fresh ground

Favorite Toppings if you choose … sometimes I add guacamole and dollops of sour cream … definitely not Spanish.
A **Romesco Sauce** is always welcomed! (recipe next page)

putting it all together

step 1: Heat oil and layer the potatoes and onions. Cook slowly—the potatoes actually "boil" in the oil. Turn mixture carefully and cook until tender—don't brown them.

step 2: Drain the mixture in a colander, retaining about 3 tablespoons of the oil on the side. Remove the scrapings from the pan—residue oil is fine—you are going to put this mixture back in the pan later.

step 3: In a bowl, beat eggs. Add salt, garlic, red pepper flakes, and olives. Add potatoes—pressing into egg mixture and let it sit for about 15 minutes.

step 4: Next, heat the 3 T of oil, you may need to add a little more—get HOT. Now, add ALL back to the pan and spread. Lower the temperature to medium and cook/brown. Get ready to do the flip to brown the other side. You may need a little oil when you flip it. I use another plate to hold the omelet in place as I turn the pan over and slide it back into the pan.

OK … if it's a mess—not to worry. Push it together … do the browning/cooking for eggs of other side … Then move it to a platter.

Cool down—serve warm or at room temperature. Of course, it can be made ahead of time.

You can cut up for appetizer servings. I just leave it all together, add your choice of toppings. For me, it's whatever my cooking muse dictates.

Romesco Sauce

yield: 2 cups

ingredients

One 15 to 16-ounce jar of roasted red bell peppers, drained, juices reserved … you will use a teaspoon at a time to thin the sauce if needed

⅓ C extra virgin olive oil

¼ C tomato paste

2 T sherry wine vinegar

2 garlic cloves, minced

1 tsp paprika

1 tsp each of kosher salt and black pepper, fresh ground

putting it all together

step 1: Combine the bell peppers, garlic, oil, paprika, tomato paste, vinegar, salt and pepper in a blender or food processor. Blend until the sauce is almost smooth. If the sauce is too thick, blend in one teaspoon of the roasted bell pepper juice at a time to thin. Cover and refrigerate.

step 2: Transfer sauce to a small bowl. The sauce can be made 1 day ahead. Cover and chill. Bring to room temperature before serving.

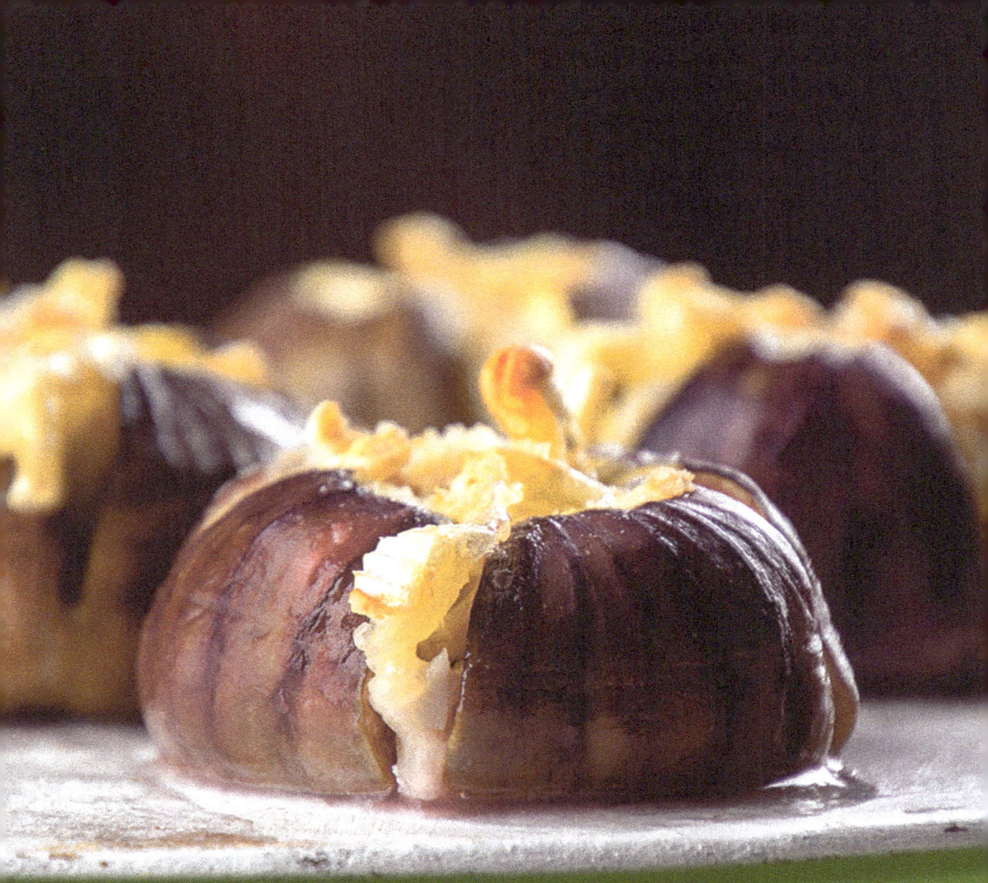

fruit

Apricot and Mango Nibbles with a Cherry on Top!

I love easy and FAST. Apricot Nibbles with a surprise cherry on top fit the bill, adding a visual lure to your appetizer offerings. Fruit is always welcomed when appetizers and snacks are offered. With dried apricots and mangos as a sturdy finger base, adding cheese and then another fruit topping, this is perfect year-round.

I like to offer both apricot and mango options at the same time. You don't have to and can let each be the solo star of your gathering.

makes: as many as you want, plan on 1 to 2 per person
prep time: less than 20 minutes | **cooking time:** none

ingredients

apricots, dried

mango slices, dried

goat cheese or Boursin cheese

sweet cherries—*fresh that you split and pit*

cherries, dried – *The juiciest dried cherries I've found are sold by Cherry Bay Orchards and are sold online. I found them on Amazon.*

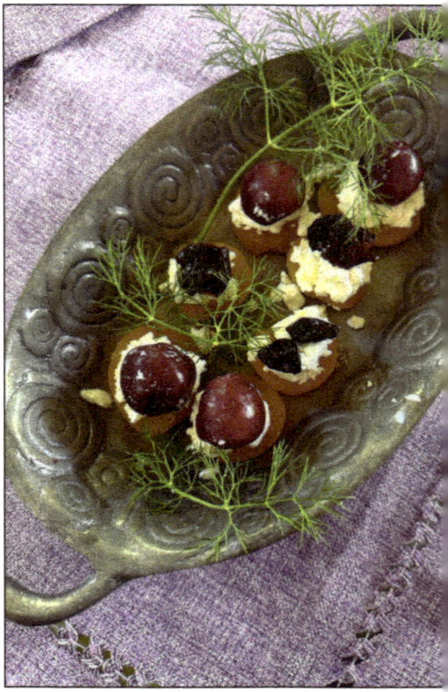

putting it all together

Roll the cheese into a small ball and place it on top of the apricot. Add the sweet cherry and gently push down. Move to your serving plate.

Dates and Bleu Cheese

I like lots of appetizers and have been known to do an entire dinner party around them ... nothing else. The variety is wide to meet any taste and/or diet restriction. Medjool dates would be my choice.

When appetizers are easy, it's a winner for anyone at the kitchen helm. If you aren't serving stuffed dates, it's time to add them to your list. What I love about them is that you can do a simple version—add a little cheese such as sharp Roquefort or Gorgonzola, an Italian bleu cheese that is a tad milder. Goat cheese also shines within a pitted date.

Your fingers will love how fast it comes together. Now you can gussy them up—add a roasted pecan on top of the cheese, a whole cashew, crunched pistachios, and TaDah! Or zest yours up ... sometimes I add a kiss of cinnamon if I'm using goat cheese or a dab of honey—so delish.

Sometimes, I serve them with half a piece of bacon wrapped around them and baked in the oven. Precook the bacon one-half to three-quarters of the way before the final bake, then wrap around the date—the oven completes the cooking. Serve hot. So delicious.

Trust me, *they will disappear quickly.*

You can serve them at room temp—I like to warm them up so that my taste buds wake up and my yum factor says hello.

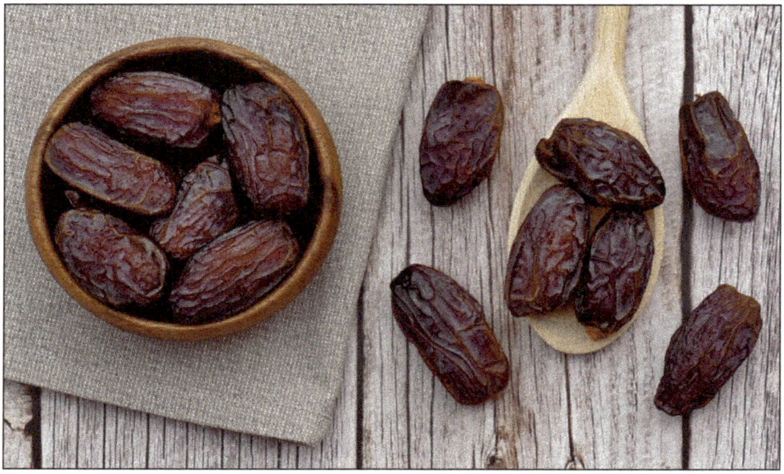

makes: 20 pieces | **preheat:** oven to 350°F and 400°F
prep time: 30 minutes | **cooking time:** 5-7 minutes

ingredients

6–8 oz. sharp bleu cheese: Roquefort, Gorgonzola, Stilton—*Other options include goat cheese.*

20 Medjool dates, pitted … *in the produce section of your grocery store.*

½ C pecans, chopped

putting it all together

step 1: Toast pecans … you want halves to place on top of the cheese filing. Bake for 5 minutes on a baking sheet.

Tip: I usually have one to two cups of these roasted and ready to go that I keep in my refrigerator—using for stuffing and salads. Half are chopped, the other a combo of halved and whole.

step 2: The dates are already split. Spread and stuff with the cheese of your choice.

step 3: Press pecan on top … serve.

Think sweet, salty, savory, and creamy, and two dates per person. Serve right away or assemble it up to 2 hours ahead, refrigerate.

Dates are the oldest cultivated fruit on Earth. The Middle East has been harvesting them for at least 6,000 years. The Greeks gave it the name we all call it. Dactylos means "finger"--the shape of this morsel.

Dates with a Zest!

Medjool dates are large dates in the "easy peasy" category that add a smidge of sweetness and a taste of caramel-like flavor to your appetizer offerings. All it takes is three ingredients.

You want the ones that are pitted, meaning the pit has been removed, and a slit in the date is ideal for stuffing of some sort.

Stuffing is usually a cheese—think Boursin, goat, or a bleu cheese. When seasonal goat cheese with cranberries surfaces in November, this adds an extra taste pop. For this one, add a sprinkle of zest once you stuff your choice of cheese ... and you are done.

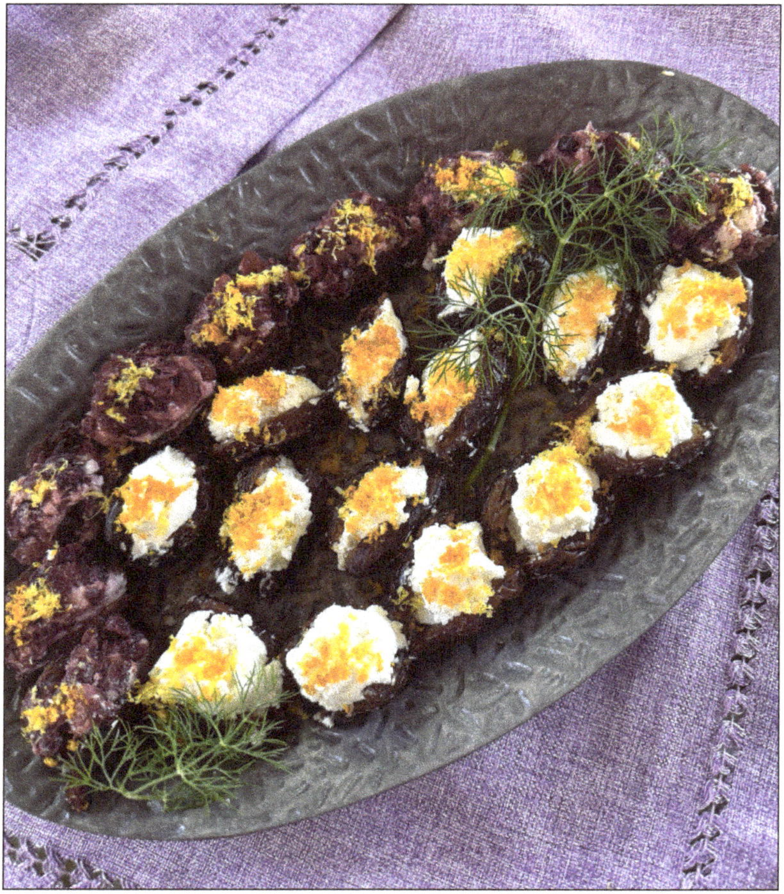

makes: 20 dates

prep time: 15-30 minutes depending on how many you make

cooking time: none

ingredients

20 Medjool dates, pitted

8 oz. cheese of your choice—Boursin, goat—plain or with cranberries, bleu cheese

1 orange, zested

1 lemon, zested

putting it all together

step 1: Remove your cheese of choice—or mix it up and have a variety—soften to room temperature. You can make ahead and refrigerate. Remember to bring them out before serving so the cheese is at room temperature.

step 2: Zest your orange. For a colorful visual variety, you could add in lemon zest, even lime—just a small amount. You want the orange to be the dominator.

step 3: Open the slit on the Medjool dates and insert cheese.

step 4: Sprinkle zested orange and lemon peels on top. Serve.

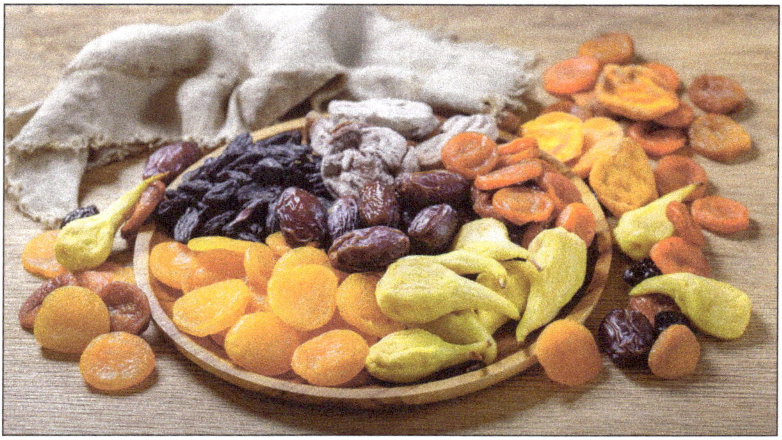

Dried Fruit Fanfare

For an easy peasy plate of a variety of fruit options, think dried fruit … fruit that's had the majority of its water removed. Always super snackable, but there is a caution: it's easy to overeat these gems. The dehydration process shrinks berries and fruits to sizes that any snacker thinks is great. It's why I like to have a few other appetizers to offer my guests, so their grazing eyes use dried fruit as almost the dessert side of what I have for them.

Your options are many, ranging from old favorites like raisins, craisins (dried cranberries), and dried apples to mangos, apricots, cherries, peach slices, bananas, and even pineapple. If you are a DIYer and have the equipment to dehydrate, go for it. My choice is to hit the grocery store and see what the bagged selections are.

makes: a large platter | **prep time:** 15 minutes | **cooking time:** none

ingredients

dried fruit—*your choice*—depending on how many types. If buying by the pound, consider this example: ½ lb of dried apricots yields about 20 pieces..

putting it all together

Let your imagination be your guide. Create your platter—have a few tong-like serving "tools" for selection picking by your guests.

Stuffed Figs with Goat Cheese and Honey

If you haven't had a fresh fig … it's time to get acquainted. My heart sister, Glenda, raved about her close encounter, and I had to get in line to try her version as an appetizer. First, I had to track down fresh ones—not dried. And fig jam isn't the substitute. I was too late in the season and had to wait. When it comes to tracking down fresh figs, start with your local grocery store locator and do the ASK—either online or on the phone. Where I live in the US, fig season is typically late May through the summer months.

Finally, success. And the wait was worth it. Prep is fairly quick. Just pipe in soft goat cheese to the center, broil a few minutes and drizzle with honey—oh my—delish! You do not want any that feel mushy at the touch—just a gentle softness.

makes: 12 figs | **preheat:** oven broiler
prep time: 15 minutes | **cooking time:** 4 minutes

ingredients

12 fresh figs

4 oz soft goat cheese or Boursin cheese

1 tsp olive oil

¼ C honey

Salt and freshly ground black pepper

putting it all together

step 1: Trim off stems of figs and cut an "X" in the top of each fig one-third of the way through. Place the figs on a parchment-lined sheet tray. If they are a little wobbly, shave a bit off the bottoms of the figs so they stand upright—this is the way you will serve them.

step 2: Place goat cheese in a plastic bag and gently massage it until softened. I then use a sandwich-sized zippered storage bag and cut a small hole in the corner of one side. You are now ready to pipe the cheese into each fig, dividing your four ounces of goat cheese evenly between the 12 figs.

step 3: Lightly brush the figs with olive oil and sprinkle with a little salt and a generous amount of freshly cracked black pepper.

step 4: Broil figs for about 4 minutes or until you can see little brown bits on the goat or Boursin cheese.

step 5: As the figs are under the broiler, separately warm the honey so it is easily pourable—not hot.

step 6: Remove figs from the oven and drizzle each one with warm honey. Serve warm or at room temperature.

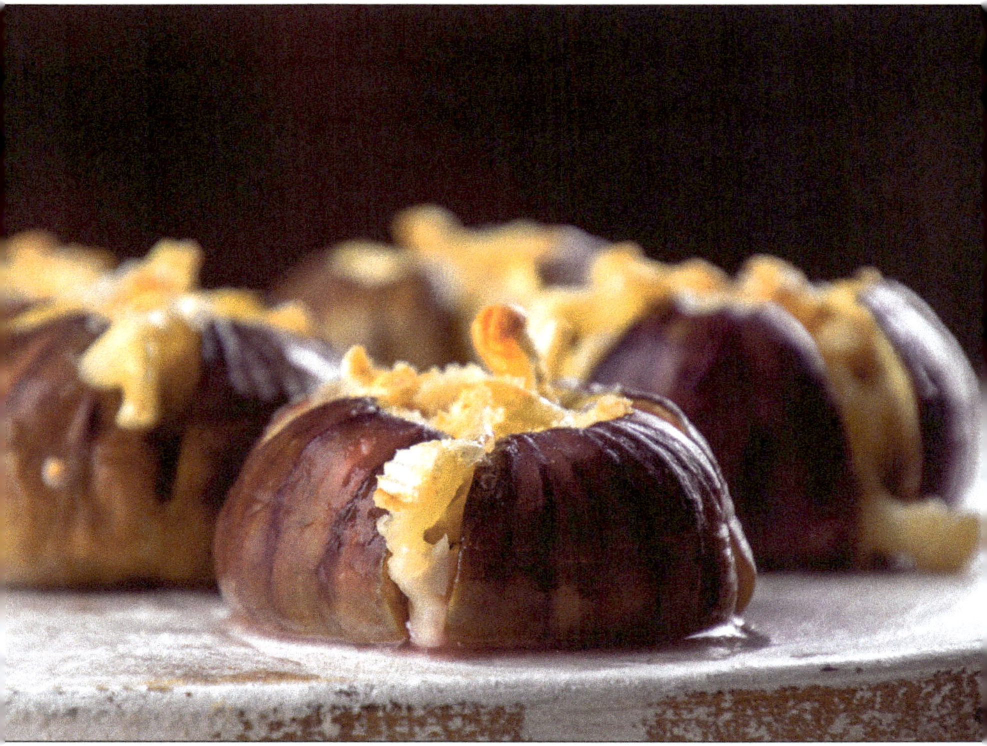

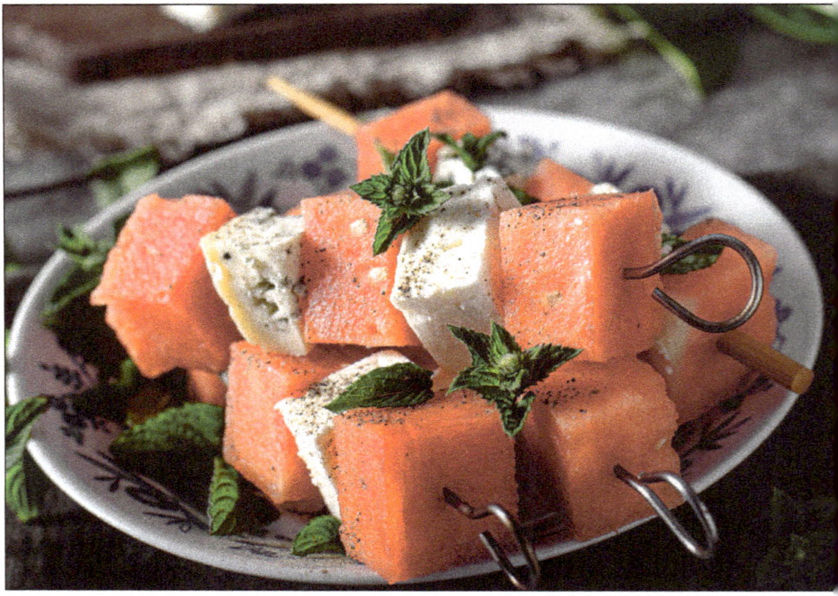

Watermelon and Feta Bites

When watermelons show up, most look for the corn on the cob and think BBQ. Oh, I can, but I'm more inclined to think salad, a light dessert, or yum, an appetizer with a salty cheese to enhance it. When I'm in a Mediterranean mood for simple food on my back deck with friends, my Watermelon and Feta Bites work. They are not heavy … almost a munching. A few of them won't fill you up. Adding a little basil or a kiss of mint, and a drizzle of balsamic vinegar, olive oil, and sprinkle of pepper perk it all up.

makes: 8 to 10 skewers

prep time: 5 minutes | **cooking time:** no cooking

ingredients

2 lbs of seedless watermelon—excluding the rind

8 oz Greek or French feta – *I find it at my local Middle Eastern market (it will be in a block)*

3 T olive oil

2–3 T balsamic vinegar—either dark or white

pepper

basil or mint

skewers, 6 inch

putting it all together

step 1: Whisk the olive oil, balsamic vinegar, and pepper together. When you get your skewers put together, you will drizzle this over the finished skewers.

step 2: Remove the rind from the watermelon, and cut into one-inch squares.

step 3: Cut the feta into ½-inch pieces.

step 4: Clip or pull medium leaves of basil and mint from stems. Rinse gently and pat dry.

step 5: Assemble your feta/watermelon skewers, starting and ending with a watermelon piece on each, and adding a basil or mint leaf on each skewer. Brush with olive oil and balsamic vinegar, and sprinkle with pepper.

step 6: Refrigerate. These can be made a few hours ahead.

Dates and Pine Nuts Crostini

Dates are usually guest favorites. I always think of pine nuts as one of the gold bars in the nut treasure chest—ideal as a pleasant surprise in a salad and a topping on an appetizer. Mix them with the easily-held crostini. They are a tasty sensation that foodie grazers go back to for another.

This is a quick appetizer to put together—I like it!

makes: 20 to 25 crostini | **preheat:** oven to 325°F
prep time: 10 minutes | **cooking time:** less than 10 minutes

ingredients

12 dates

½ C pine nuts, toasted … *I do 325°F oven for about 4 minutes or dry roast in skillet for a few minutes. Stay close—a golden light brown is the goal.*

⅓ C red wine … *a blended red works fine*

¼ C honey … *or a tad more*

¼ tsp garlic powder

baguette, sliced and toasted in oven with olive oil

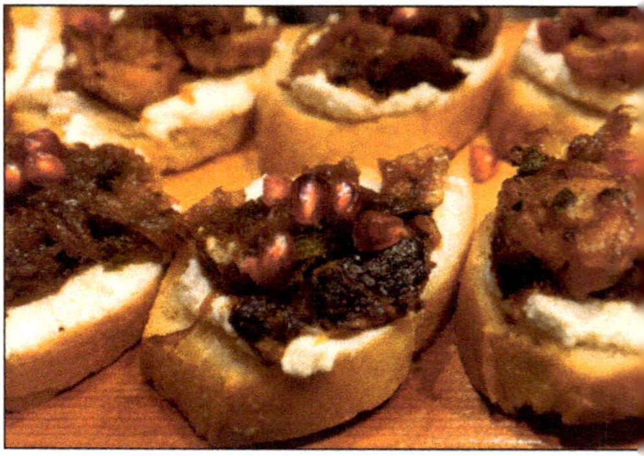

putting it all together

step 1: Slice baguettes. Mix olive oil and garlic powder, then spread on top of baguettes. Bake until a touch of tan shows—no more than 6 minutes. At the same time, you can do the pine nuts—watch closely, the pine nuts brown quickly.

step 2: Chop dates—add to a pan on stove top with pine nuts, honey, and wine—cook about 5 minutes.

step 3: Spread warm on a toasted baguette—yummy!

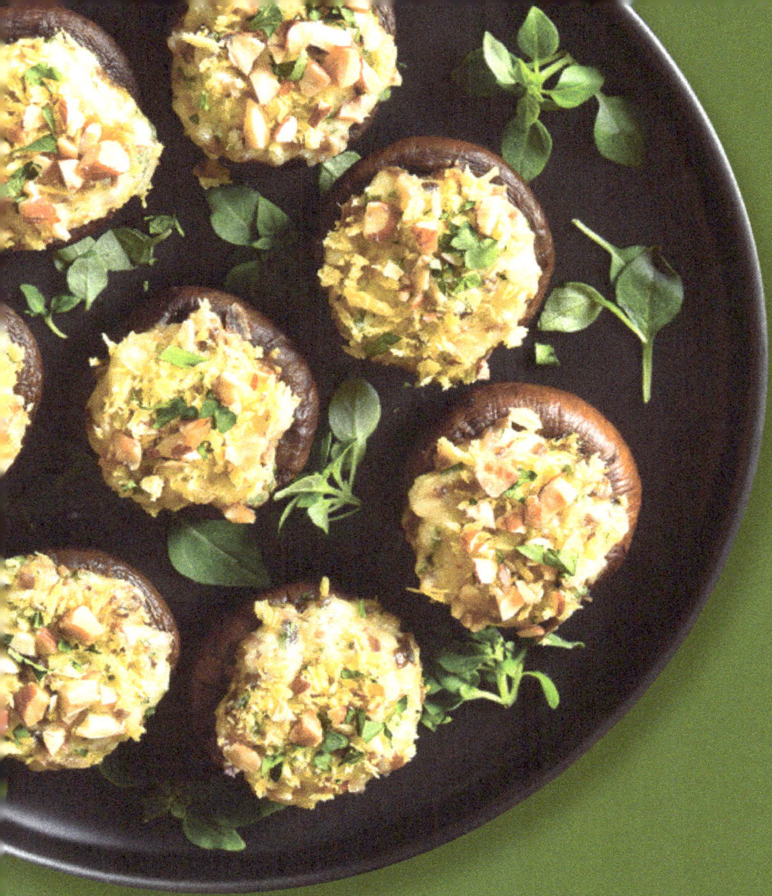

prosciutto, bacon, and ham

Bacon and Cheddar Cheese Potato Rounds

For a heavier appetizer, Bacon and Cheese Potato Rounds are a hit with any hungry crowd. This is an ideal add when you want to offer a variety—some light, others filling. I've included them when I do an appetizer meal with a side salad.

makes: 20 rounds | **preheat:** over to 400°F
prep time: 15 minutes | **cooking time:** 35 minutes

ingredients

4 medium baking potatoes … cut into ¼ to ⅜-inch slices, leave skins on

½ C butter, melted

1½ C cheddar cheese, grated

10 slices of bacon, cooked and crumbled

½ C chopped green onions

Sour cream for final topping option to dab on each

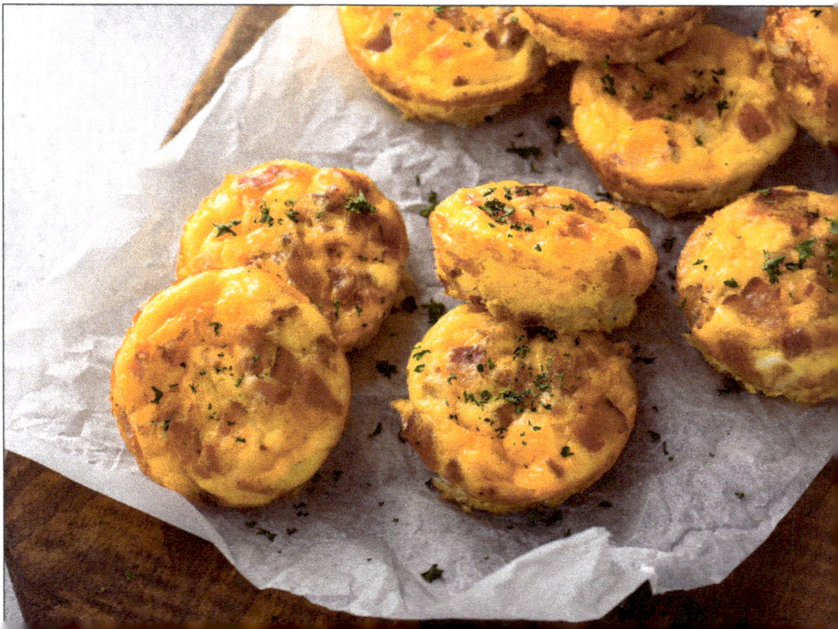

putting it all together

step 1: Line a baking sheet with parchment paper.

step 2: Generously brush both sides of sliced potatoes with melted butter and place on a baking sheet. I confess … I've dipped the entire slice into the butter and skipped the brushing. Add a small sprinkling of salt and pepper. Place on baking sheet.

step 3: Bake for 15 minutes and flip them. Continue baking until lightly browned and tender when you poke with a knife or fork … about another 15-20 minutes.

step 4: Remove from oven and top with grated cheddar cheese, crumbled bacon, and cut green onions. Bake about 3-4 more minutes.

step 5: Serve immediately. Warm as finger food or on a small plate with a fork. Include a side bowl of sour cream, queso, or even horseradish sauce for an added topping.

Bacon Lover's Bow Tie Crackers

Appetizers scream for crackers … dress yours up with a little snap, sass, and salt. Bacon belongs somewhere on your table spread … combine all and add a homemade dip with two or three of the soft herbs of your choice. The visual pulls your guests in … their fingers will do the walking toward your serving dish. I promise you … these disappear. The herbs you add are to your taste—you're the host.

makes: 48 Bow Tie Crackers | **preheat:** oven to 250°F
prep time: 10 minutes | **cooking time:** 90 minutes

ingredients

48 Club Crackers

1 lb of bacon … *regular slices, cut in half lengthwise*

herbs … basil, cilantro, dill, mint, or parsley … select two or three to chop up for dip

ingredients for dip

6 T herbs, chopped finely: basil, cilantro, dill, mint, or parsley—*select two or three to chop up for dip*

½ C mayonnaise

1 C sour cream

1 tsp onion powder

½ tsp garlic salt

½ tsp pepper

putting it all together

step 1: Wrap bacon around crackers. Bake slowly.

putting the dip together

step 1: Mix mayonnaise, sour cream, onion powder, garlic salt, and pepper.

step 2: Chill for at least two hours.

step 3: Serve dip with cooled Bow Tie Crackers.

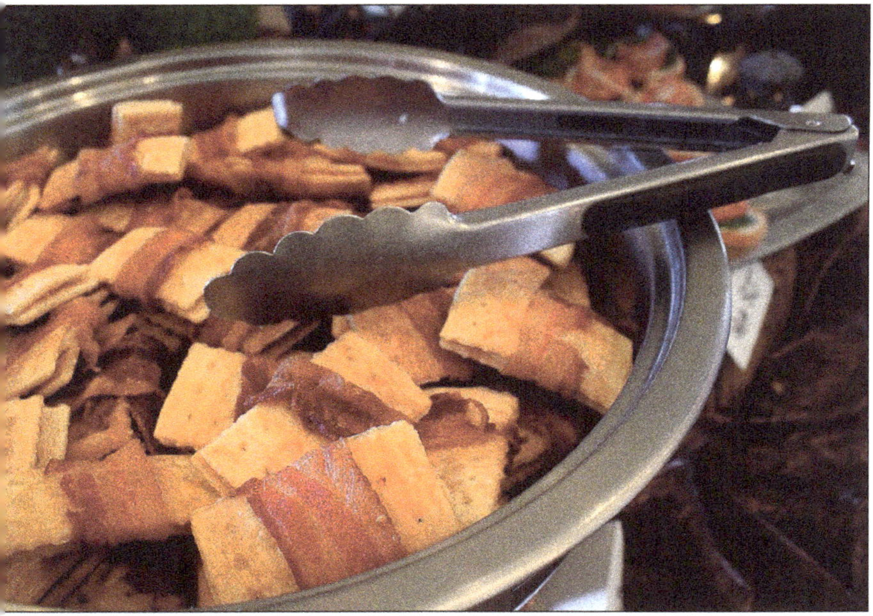

Brie, Pear, and Prosciutto Skewers

These Brie and pear skewers topped with prosciutto are quick and easy, bringing a sweet and savory appetizer that your guests will love! You have three stars here: cheese, pears, and prosciutto. Think of two cheese possibilities: Brie and bleu. Backup would be a feta or goat. The pears you use should give slightly at the neck with the body of pear firmer—not hard. The prosciutto should be thin and rolled as the topper.

You can make ahead … but keep your time within two hours of serving. Refrigerate of course, and remove 30 minutes before serving, so the cheese comes to room temperature.

makes: 8 skewers

prep time: 20 minutes | **cooking time:** none

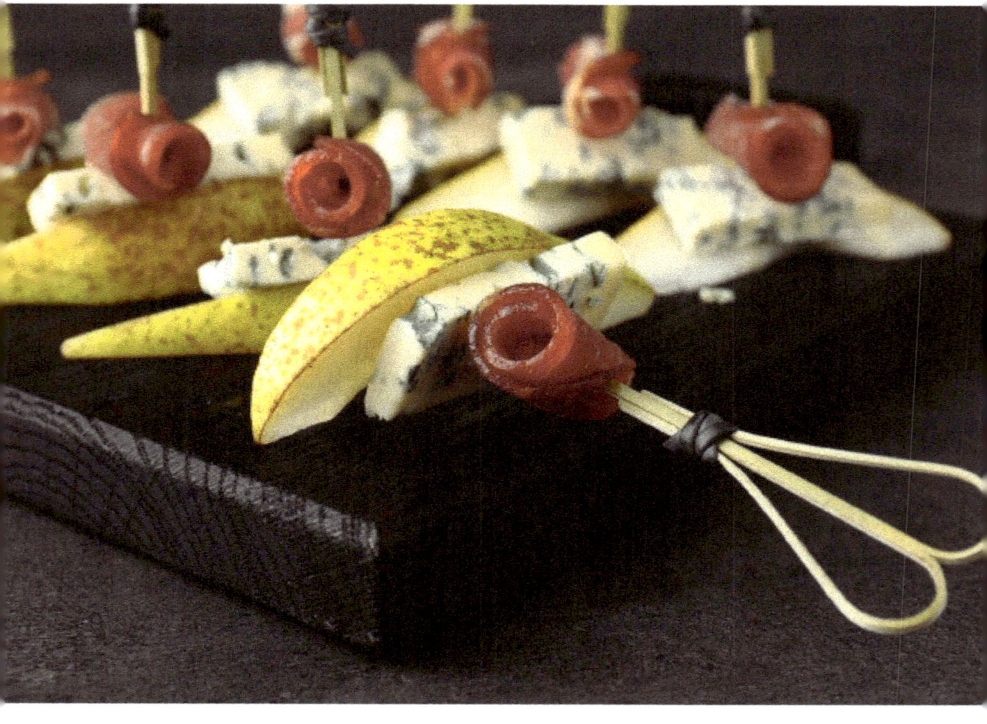

ingredients

2 pears, Bosc or Bartlett, leave skin on

8 oz Brie cheese … or bleu cheese, goat, or feta

½ C pecans, chopped

balsamic vinegar

skewers, short

putting it all together

step 1: Slice pears into quarters and remove seeds and stem. Cut quarters into slices that will become the base of your skewer. If slicing the pear in advance, dip the slices in a 1:1 mixture of water and lemon juice to slow the browning/oxidation process.

step 2: Cut Brie cheese into similar-sized slices, slightly smaller. Press a small amount of the chopped pecans into the brie for a surprise taste.

step 3: Top with the prosciutto that you have rolled.

step 4: Take a 4 to 6 inch skewer and thread the pear, cheese, and then prosciutto. Repeat until all cheese and pears are used up.

step 5: Once all skewers are on the platter, drizzle balsamic vinegar over them.

Brussels Sprouts with Bacon Wrap

Brussels sprouts used to be the vegetable most ignored. With added flavorings and bacon, that will easily disappear. It is best to roast them together on a sheet pan, wrapping the sprout with the bacon along with a kiss of honey and the added zing of the Parmesan crisps. The fat creates a crispy crunch.

This one will become a repeat for you and your guests.

makes: 12 wraps | **preheat:** oven to 400°F
prep time: 20 minutes | **cooking time:** 30 minutes

ingredients

1 lb Brussels sprouts, halved if large

1 lb bacon—*medium, never thick*

3 T olive oil

1 T honey

1 pinch each kosher salt and cracked black pepper

½ C Parmesan

½ C Parmesan crisps, crushed

ingredients for Ranch Dressing

½ C sour cream or Greek yogurt-plain

⅓ C buttermilk*

1 T chives, dried

1 tsp dill, dried

½ tsp garlic powder

½ tsp onion powder

kosher salt and cracked black pepper to taste

**Buttermilk substitute:* combine 1½ tsp of lemon juice or white vinegar with enough milk to equal one-half cup. Stir and sit for 5-10 minutes until it slightly thickens and curdles. It will be good for up to two weeks.

putting it all together

step 1: Make **Ranch Dressing** (page 94) for dipping and refrigerate until you are ready to use. Or, create dressing from a packaged mix or use ready-made salad dressing.

step 2: Preheat the oven to 400°F. Halve the Brussels sprouts.

step 2: Trim any stems from the Brussels sprouts. Parboil (blanching) them for 3-4 minutes in boiling water. This will expedite your cooking time in the oven. Immediately transfer to ice water to stop cooking and retain green color. Drain and dry.

step 4: Trim the white ends of the bacon. Discard. Cut the bacon strips into halves or thirds. You want it to wrap around the halved Brussels sprout.

step 5: Use a rimmed baking sheet, toss together the dried Brussels sprouts, olive oil, honey, and a pinch each of salt and pepper. Add the Parmesan. IF you also add the Parmesan crisps from the grocery store, crumble and mix in to your toss.

step 6: Wrap each sprout in bacon, placing each seam side down on the baking sheet. If a halved sprout, the halved side down. Roast the Brussels sprouts on the lower oven rack until browned, 20 minutes. Flip and cook another 5-10 minutes, until browned and crisp.

Serve the warm sprouts with ranch on the side.

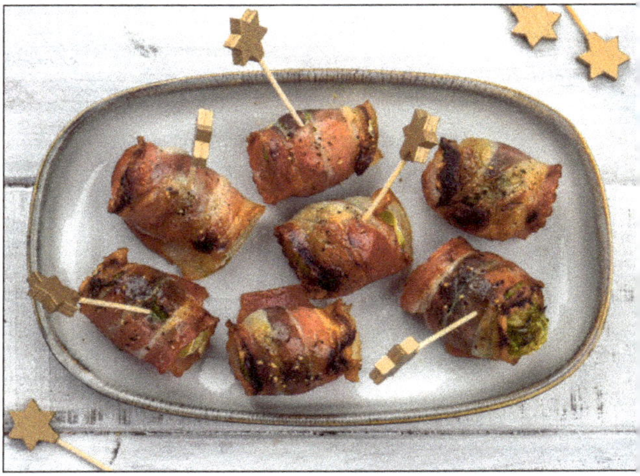

Dates Stuffed with Bacon and Bleu Cheese

I like lots of appetizers and have been known to do an entire dinner party around them … nothing else. The variety is wide to meet any taste and/or diet restriction. Medjools would be my date choice.

When appetizers are easy, it's a winner for anyone at the kitchen helm. If you aren't serving stuffed dates, it's time to add them to your list. What I love about them is that you can do a simple version—add a little cheese such as sharp Roquefort or Gorgonzola, an Italian bleu cheese that is a tad milder. Goat cheese also shines within a pitted date.

Your fingers will love how fast it comes together. Now you can gussy them up—add a roasted pecan on top of the cheese, a whole cashew, crunched pistachios, and TaDah! Or zest yours up … sometimes I add a kiss of cinnamon if I'm using goat cheese or a dab of honey—so delish.

Sometimes, I serve them with half a piece of bacon wrapped around them and baked in the oven. Precook the bacon one-half to three-quarters of the way before the final bake, then wrap around the date—the oven completes the cooking. Serve hot. So delicious.

Trust me, they will disappear quickly.

You can serve them at room temp—I like to warm them up so that my taste buds wake up and my yum factor says hello.

makes: makes 20 dates | **preheat:** over to 350°F and then 400°F
prep time: 30 minutes | **cooking time:** 5-7 minutes

ingredients

¾ lb. sharp bleu cheese …. Roquefort, Gorgonzola, Stilton—*Other options include goat cheese.*

20 Medjool dates—*in the produce section of your grocery store*

1 lb. bacon

½ C pecans, chopped

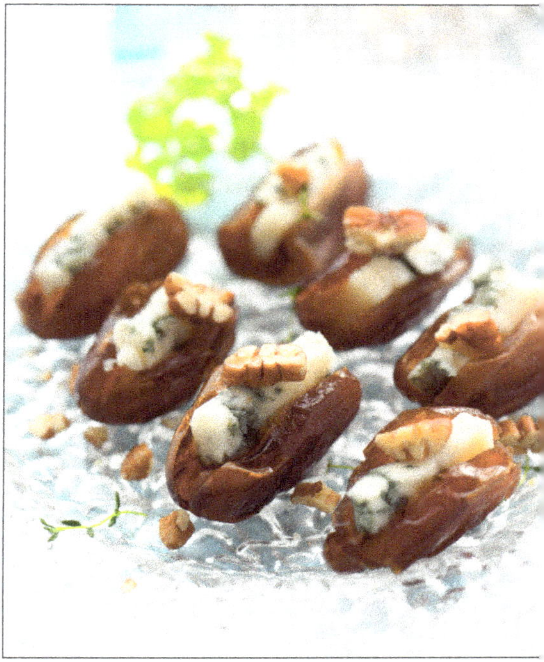

putting it all together

step 1: Toast pecans … you want halves to place on top of the cheese filing. 350°F for 5 minutes on a baking sheet.

step 3: Precook bacon in a skillet (usually half a slice) to half to three-fourths done—you want it limp to wrap around the date. This will take a few minutes. Drain.

step 3: Stuff dates, wrap bacon around each one, and bake at 400°F for 7 minutes … serve.

Think sweet, salty, savory, and creamy, and two dates per person. Serve right away or assemble it up to 2 hours ahead, refrigerate. Bring bacon-stuffed dates to room temperature for 20-30 minutes before serving.

Farro Mediterranean Summer Affair

Discover FARRO, used in many Mediterranean dishes. It's hearty and when I make it for friends, there are no leftovers, or they take it home. Whatever they can get from me.

Want full Italian? Substitute a rotini-type pasta for the farro.

What I like about this dish is that it's got many roles: appetizer, salad, or a side. I'm a firm believer in having a variety of small plates that my friends and guests can mix and match. Let them choose "one of" or scoop your treat onto a small plate that is enjoyed in a few bites. My Farro Mediterranean Summer Affair is perfect for this.

Mix in veggies, feta cheese, and Italian meats. Your salad can be a side or a main course. Generously toss it with a homemade dressing, or do the cheat: get the bottled Newman's Italian Dressing or the Olive Garden Dressing that Costco carries. Either works well.

What I love … this is such an easy, Mediterranean salad recipe that has lots of vitamins with the farro grain. My cheat: I cook the farro in a rice cooker, so I don't have to monitor cooking process. Then, I can chop the other ingredients and mix with veggies and cheese when the farro is done. I do it all in less than 25 minutes. I make a generous amount of salad dressing since it gets soaked up once it is chilled in the refrigerator. And I do it in the morning, so all the ingredients can hang out to meld flavors before serving later.

makes: 30, ½ cup servings | **prep time:** 25 minutes
cooking time: 20 minutes for farro or until done

ingredients

1 lb box of farro per instructions … *if you want to perk up the water it's cooking in, add one generous teaspoon of Better Than Bouilion base, beef, chicken, or vegetable*

7 oz salami -I use thick and thin … just cut it up

8-10 oz feta cheese, cut up

1 C grape tomatoes, sliced in half

½–1 C Parmesan cheese

6 mini-cucumbers, cut up
(much crisper than regular cucumbers)

1 C diced celery

1 C Kalamata olives, cut in half *(my favorite olive)*

1–2 avocados, cut up

½ red onion, diced

½ C basil, cut in ribbons

1-2 red, orange, or yellow bell peppers, diced

ingredients for Newman's homemade salad dressing

makes: 3 cups

2 C of virgin olive oil

3-4 oz of red wine vinegar, *if you like it really tart, or balsamic vinegar if you like it sweeter—why not both, blend the two?*

2-3 T of Dijon mustard—Grey Poupon, *which is sharp-flavored or even a whole grain variety that features crushed mustard seed for texture.*

1 tsp celery seeds

salt to taste, approximately 1-2 tsp

1-2 tsp pepper

putting it all together

Start by bringing a large pot of water to a boil. Cook farro according to package instruction … OR in rice cooker … water, farro, salt, cover and push button. It stops when the liquid is absorbed.

step 1: Make sure to generously salt your water before you cook the farro in it! Drain and set aside, or use a rice cooker—my preference.

step 2: Cut the vegetables, meats, and cheese into small cubes.

step 3: Toss the cooked farro with the dressing and add the vegetables first and then the salami and cheeses. Top with fresh Parmesan cheese and basil.

step 5: Cover and refrigerate until ready to serve. This is an ideal make-ahead.

Garnish option: fresh basil (cut into ribbons)

putting the dressing together

Make the dressing in a blender or whisk in a bowl by combining all of the ingredients. Taste for seasonings and add more salt and pepper as needed. You will use at least one cup of it … For the "cheat," get a bottle of store-bought Newman's Salad Dressing or Olive Garden Dressing.

Tip: If you make the dressing ahead of time, cover/add a lid and do not refrigerate! When ready to use, shake the heck out of it before serving.

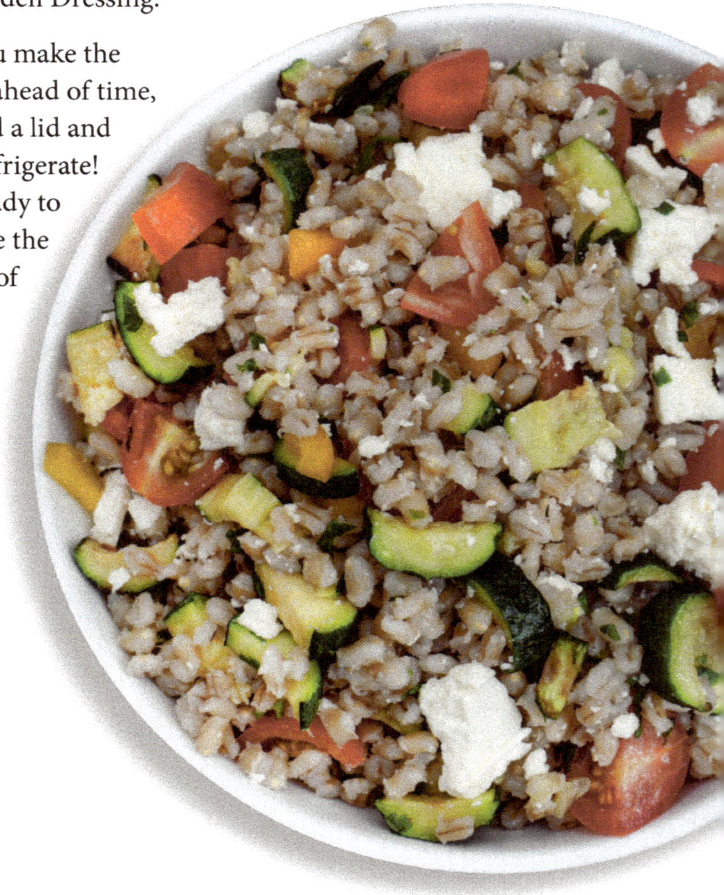

Prosciutto and Cream Cheese-Stuffed Mushrooms

If you are into mushroom appetizers, this one is a savory, impressive bite that comes together in under 30 minutes and can be prepped in advance. All good news when a gathering is imminent. I like the add of the prosciutto with the smoothness of the cream cheese that blends quickly in your oven when baking. Plus, the tarragon is a sweet, anise, and slightly peppery add. Tarragon can overpower, so stick with the ¼ tsp recommended.

makes: 16 to 20 mushrooms | **preheat:** oven to 350°F
prep time: 15 minutes | **cooking time:** 20 minutes

ingredients

16-20 cremini/button mushrooms

4 oz softened cream cheese

3 T chopped prosciutto

1 T Dijon mustard

½ C panko breadcrumbs

¼ tsp dried tarragon

1 lemon, zested

butter

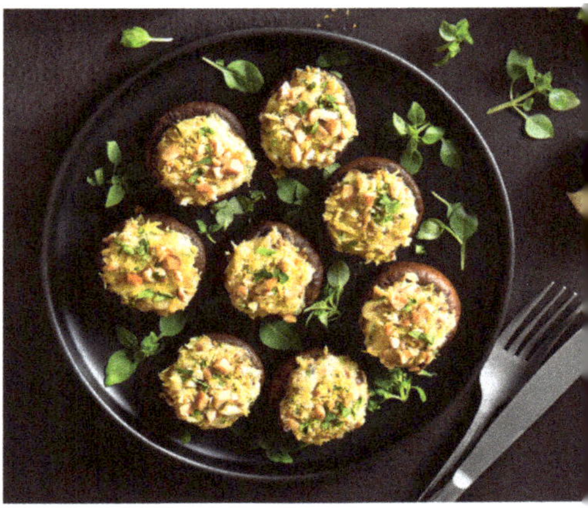

putting it all together

step 1: Pop out stems and chop them finely. Sauté the stems and prosciutto in butter for 5-6 minutes.

step 2: Remove from heat and stir in the cream cheese, tarragon, Dijon, bread crumbs, and lemon zest.

step 3: Spoon the mixture into mushroom caps and bake at 350°F for 20 minutes.

Prosciutto, Pear, and Cheese Wraps … think Brie or Gorgonzola

Prosciutto is ham—a very thin ham. It is flavorful, salty, and has a sweet taste. Some prosciutto varieties are seasoned with spices and herbs like black pepper and garlic. There are two types: prosciutto cotto, *which is cooked, and* prosciutto crudo, *which is uncooked, yet cured.*

Experiment with it. It goes well with melons—honeydew is one of my favorites. It is great to wrap around other food, like asparagus, or quickly fry and crumble it, adding it to your salads or eggs.

makes: 8 to 10 wraps
prep time: 20–30 minutes | **cooking time:** none

ingredients

5 slices of prosciutto (about 3 oz)

2 ripe pears, cored and sliced into 10 pieces

8 oz Gorgonzola or Brie

arugula, small bunch

honey for drizzle

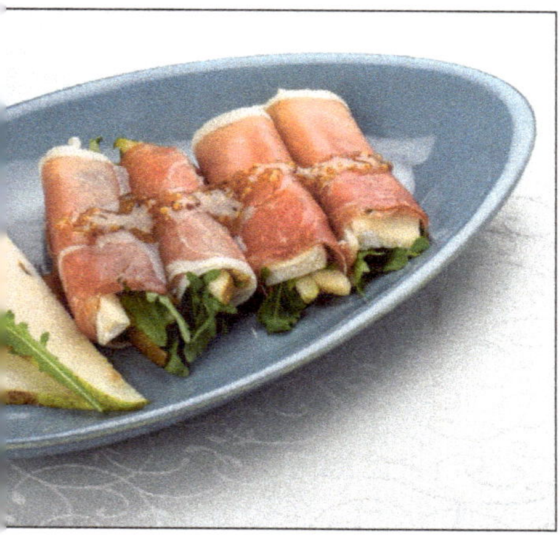

putting it all together

step 1: Create 10 pieces of ham by cutting the original 5 in half crosswise.

step 2: On each piece, lay two pieces of pear and two of the cheese. Add a small amount of the arugula. Let a little stick out at the ends.

step 3: Roll tightly. If long, cut in half to make more for your platter. Drizzle with honey in the middle of each.

Hawaiian Bruschetta

Outdoor times call for all things bruschetta. It's one of the ideal nibbles that comes together quickly. Rarely do you find pineapple in them … and why not? Oh, there's a drip factor … but here's the plus. The toasted baguette pieces welcome drips.

makes: 35 to 40 bruschetta | **preheat:** oven to 350°F
prep time: 20 minutes | **cooking time:** 8 minutes

ingredients

1-2 baguettes, sliced and toasted

3 slices of ham, cut into small pieces

1 C of combined cheeses: mozzarella, shredded, and Parmesan, grated

1 C olive oil

1 pineapple, canned, diced

1 C mango, ripe and firm

1 C avocado, chopped

½ C strawberries, sliced

½ C red onion, finely chopped

1 lime

2 garlic cloves, diced

parsley, chopped

4 T butter

putting it all together

step 1: You have two components—the sliced baguette that needs the cheesy garlic butter added to it and baked. And the chopping and combining of the fruits and other ingredients.

step 2: Do the fruit first so it chills for an hour. Then the baguette with baked cheeses. When the baguettes slices have cooled, dollop with one tablespoon of the fruit combo salsa or you can let your guests add the amount to the baked baguette slice. Serve immediately.

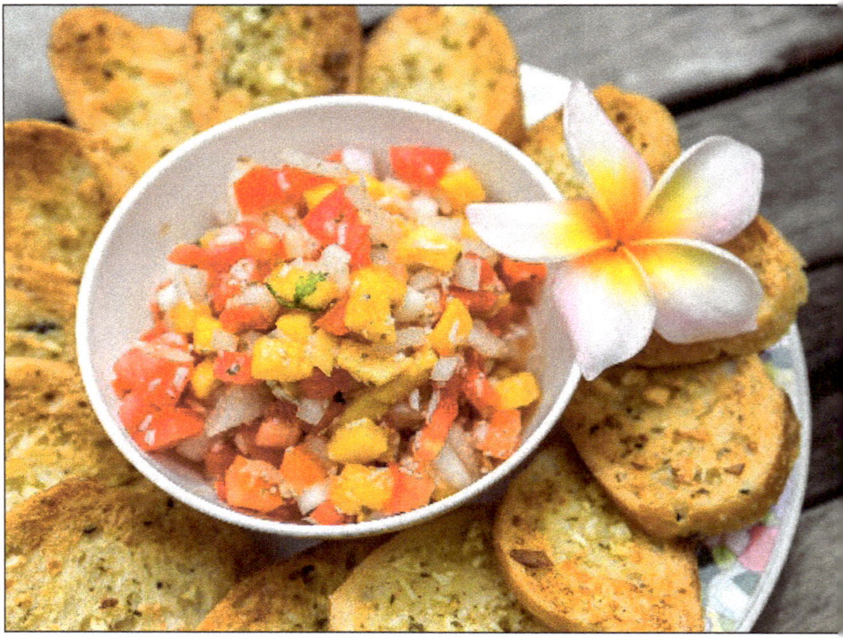

Cheesy Garlic Butter Spread

4 T butter, unsalted and softened

2 garlic cloves, chopped

pinch of dry parsley

salt and pepper — *not much*

1 C total of grated mozzarella and Parmesan cheeses, combined

step 1: Soften butter to room temp. In mixing bowl, put all the other ingredients together and stir until seasonings are mixed well. Taste and adjust seasoning if needed. Store at cool room temperature until needed or keep in chiller if doing ahead of time.

step 2: Spread on sliced baguette pieces. Bake 6 to 8 minutes. Set aside to add fruit salsa topping.

Avocado, Mango, Pineapple, Strawberry Salsa Topping

1 pineapple, canned, diced

2 mangos, diced

1 C strawberries, diced

2 C avocados, diced

2 shallots, diced

½ C red onion, chopped

2 garlic cloves, minced

3 slices of ham, chopped

salt and pepper

1 lime, juiced

step 1: Combine all ingredients and mix in a bowl. Salt and pepper to taste. Pour line juice over ingredients. Toss to coat well and chill for an hour.

step 2: Assemble in a bowl and serve with bruschetta slices. This is a "juicy" mix. Let your guests mound how much they want. on each piece.

Puff Pastry Ham and Cheese Pinwheels

I like it when tasty is easy to do. These ham and cheese pinwheels are "light" yet filling. They look like they took time to create … but no. There is no dough making—you will use already made puff pastry … found at the grocery store. This will eliminate a few hours of kitchen time.

makes: 10 to 15 pinwheels | **preheat:** oven to 375°F
prep time: 10 minutes | **cooking time:** 20-25 minutes

ingredients

cooking spray

1½ C Gruyère cheese, grated (about 6 oz)

½ C onion, finely chopped—*I use Vidalia or Maui*

2 T butter for sautéing onion

all-purpose flour, for the counter work surface

1 sheet puff pastry (from a 17.3-oz package), thawed

3 T Dijon mustard

5 oz deli ham thinly sliced—*use your favorite. I like honey, maple, and peppered ham best.*

black pepper, fresh ground

Chives, fresh and chopped for garnish, if desired

putting it all together

step 1: Preheat oven to 375°F. Lightly grease a large, parchment paper–lined rimmed baking sheet.

step 2: Grate cheese and set aside. Sauté onion in butter until translucent.

step 3: On a floured work surface, roll puff pastry into a 12x16-inch rectangle. Top with the Dijon mustard, spreading completely to the edges. Next, top with ham, scatter onions, then the cheese. Season with pepper—not necessary if you are using pepper ham.

step 4: Get ready to roll the filled pastry into a log. Do not roll loosely. Starting at one short end, tightly roll up.

step 5: Cut log into ½-inch thick pieces; transfer to the prepared parchment- lined baking sheet. Clear a space in your freezer to slip the pan in. Freeze 5 minutes.

step 6: Bake until golden brown, 20-25 minutes. Remove from oven and top with chives. Serve warm or at room temperature.

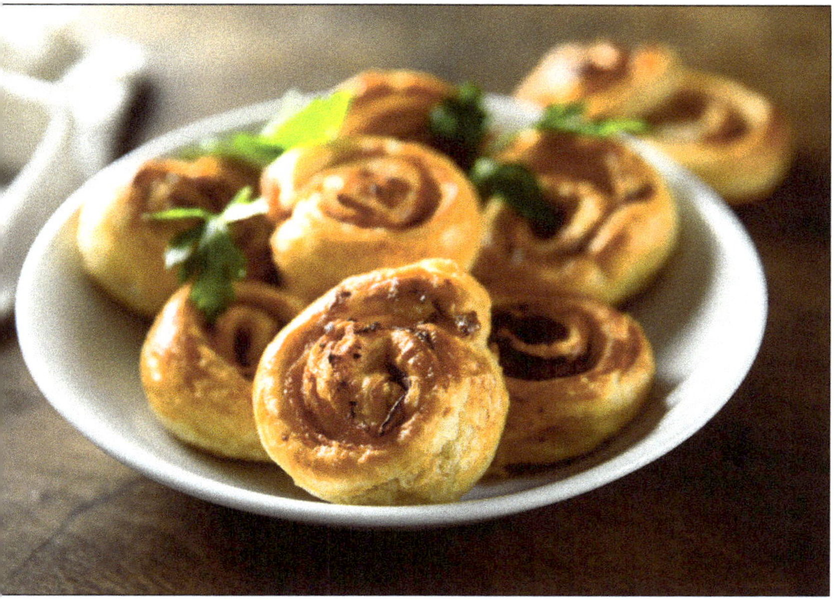

What you create and serve your friends

is your nest egg.

Fun and delicious food choices are

the investments that have the best of returns.

— Judith Briles

seafood

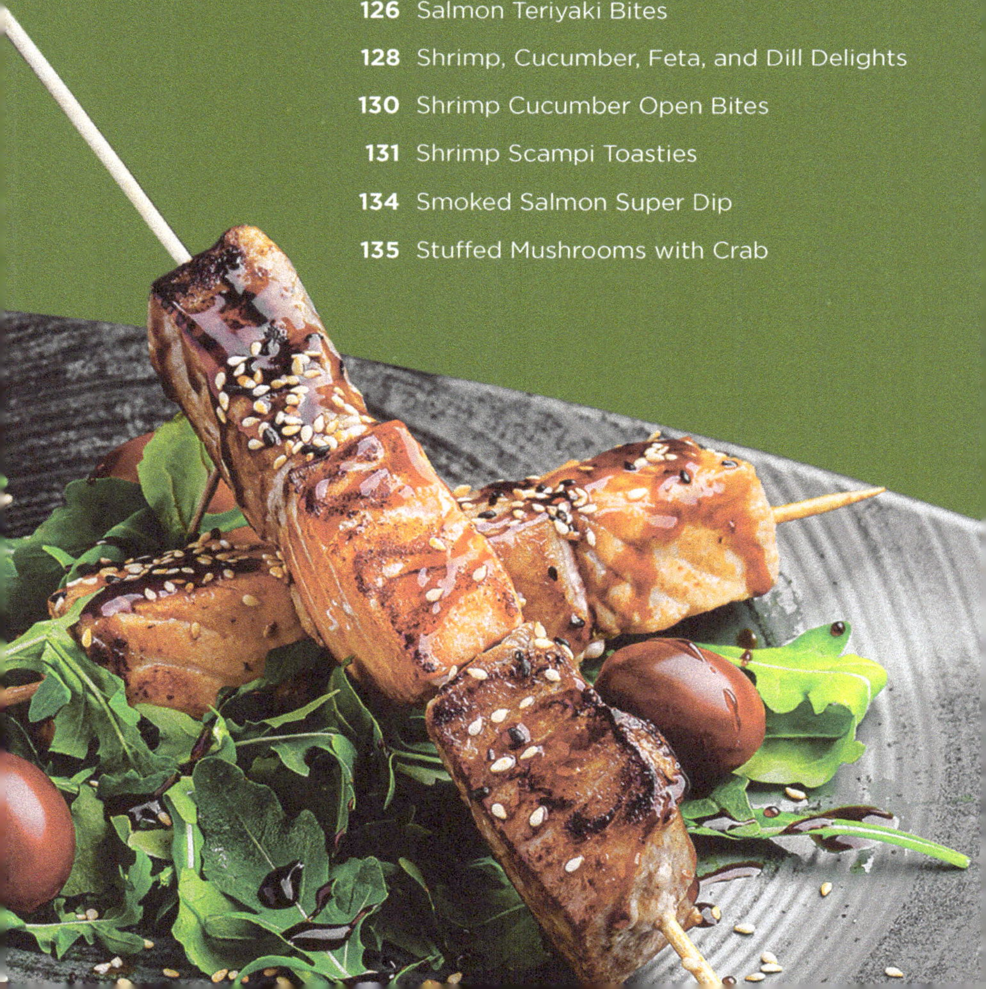

Crab Cakes Are Always a Star

When I have multiple offerings and a crab cake tray is one on them … it's the one that is emptied first. I have been serving them for decades and are routinely asked for. Jumbo lump crab is my choice … not the smaller blue crab that for me, disappears when other ingredients are added to the cake creation. I like to see that crab is the star ingredient in each one.

Crab cakes welcome a dip—sometimes I have one … sometimes a few. This is your choice time—do yourself a favor and have them made ahead.

makes: 2½ to 3 dozen for bite-sized. *Before you start putting it all together, I would make the* **Horseradish Sauce** *(page 111) and* **Chili Lime Aoili Sauce** *(page 112).*

preheat: oven to 375°F | **prep time:** 30 minutes

cooking time: 15–20 minutes or pan-fry them for about 6-8 minutes total

ingredients

12 oz lump crab—*I use Phillips*

panko (or crumbs from 2 slices of white bread, without crusts)

1 T Dijon mustard

1 tsp Worcestershire sauce

2 tsp Old Bay seasoning

1 shallot, large, minced

2 eggs, lightly beaten

zest from one lemon

horseradish—*I use Reese's or Bookbinder's*

sea salt and pepper for taste

3–4 T canola oil or butter for frying

option: 1 T cilantro, finely chopped

putting it all together

step 1: Decide on a sauce for your crab cakes—you definitely want one. I've got two below to choose from or offer both. Each takes about three minutes to put together. Suggest you refrigerate for 30 minutes.

step 2: Use two medium to large bowls. In one, gently mix your crab with your panko or breadcrumbs—set aside. In the other, mix everything else.

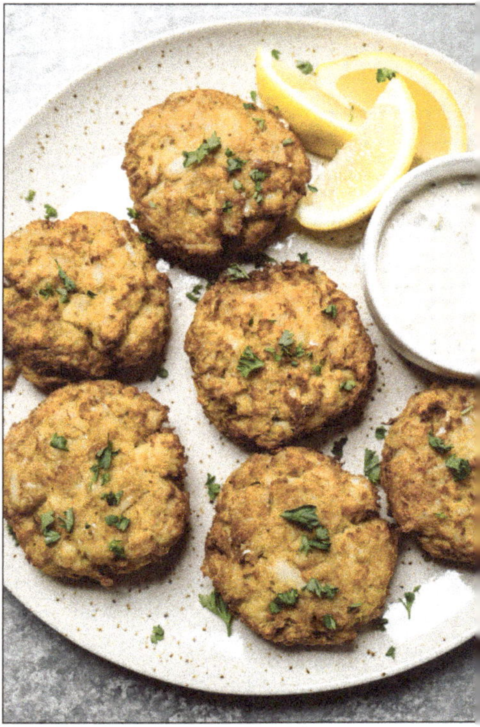

step 3: Use your hands to shape each crab cake. Mini bites are 1½ tablespoons.

step 4: If baking, preheat your oven. I like to use a large baking sheet with parchment paper as I create the cake patties and then moving it into the oven for final stage.

For frying, do in batches in either canola oil or butter—meaning this is not done on high heat—gentle golden browning.

step 5: After cooking, transfer to paper towels to absorb butter/oil for "a few minutes.

Definitely serve them warm with a sauce.

Horseradish Sauce

This creamy horseradish sauce can be used with your crab cakes. Your prep time is less than 3 minutes. It isn't overly pungent and won't mask the flavors of the crab. If you are looking for "more kick" … add more horseradish to taste.

ingredients

makes: 1 cup

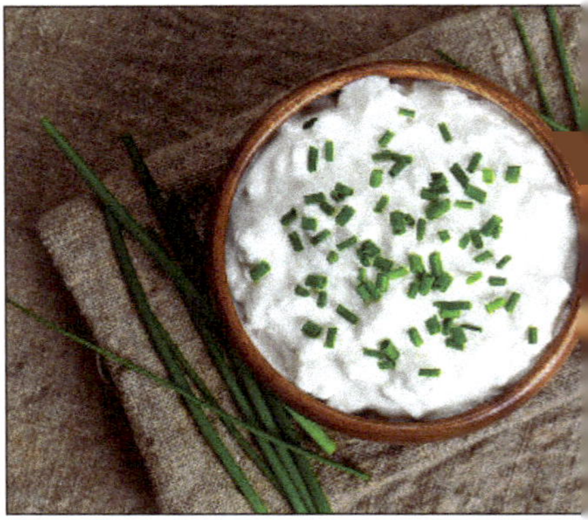

½ C sour cream

2 T prepared horseradish, drained—*check your grocery store*

2 T mayonnaise

1 tsp apple cider vinegar

¼ tsp sea salt

⅛ tsp black pepper

1 T chives, finely chopped

putting it all together

Chop and mix all except chives. Done. Refrigerate until serving in a favorite small bowl. Sprinkle chives on top.

Chili Lime Aioli Sauce

Add a creamy, zesty, and slightly spicy condiment to your mix.

makes: ½ cup

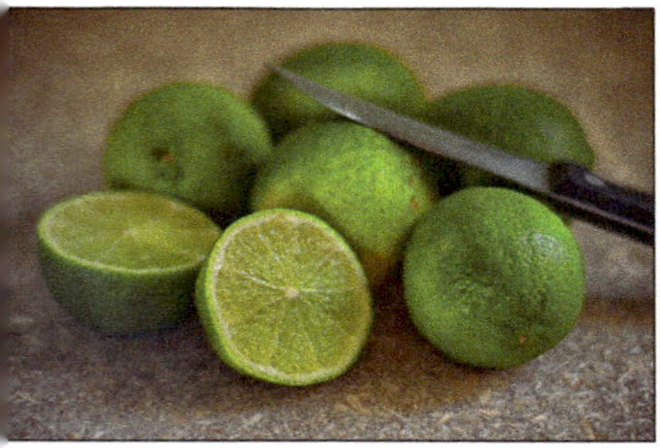

ingredients

½ C mayonnaise

zest from one lime plus 2 tsp juice

1 tsp chili powder or flavor to taste with a hot sauce—*I use Cholula*

½ tsp smoked paprika

½ tsp garlic powder

pinch of sea salt

putting it all together

Whisk all in a bowl until smooth. Make ahead and refrigerate to let the flavors meld.

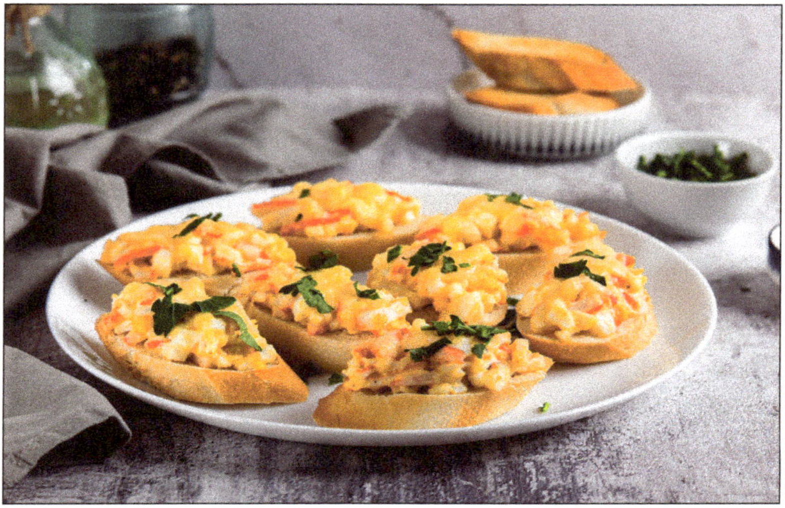

Crab Lovers' Cheesy Herb Bites

Crab can easily be served hot or cold when it comes to appetizers … meaning right out of the oven or refrigerator. When either type goes to room temperature, they lose their pop. When the English muffin or baguette slice is toasted just right, the added "crunch" is perfect.

My little Crab Lovers' Cheesy Herb Bites are easy to assemble. My preference is to use mini English muffins or a sliced baguette. For mini English muffins, Wolfermans.com is the order spot.

makes: 20 bites | **preheat:** oven to 400°F
prep time: 15 minutes | **cooking time:** 18 minutes

Ingredients

½ C butter, softened

½ tsp garlic powder

½ tsp paprika

2 T mayonnaise

1 5.3 oz Boursin garlic and herb cheese spread

8 oz lump crab—*I use Phillips*

1 package mini English muffins—*I use Wolferman's or a baguette, sliced.*

Garnish with favorite herb after removing from oven.

If you can't find the mini muffins, use regular—you will cut them into quarters after baking. Or slice a baguette, and spread on your crab mixture, then bake.

Putting it all together

step 1: Mix the first 5 ingredients together.

step 2: Gently, add in the lump crab. Do not over mix.

step 3: Slice muffins in half horizontally or slice a baguette.

step 4: Spread with the Boursin/crab mixture.

step 5: Bake and brown … watch carefully to avoid burning.

step 6: If using a regular size muffins, cut each muffin half into quarters when cool enough to handle.

step 7: Serve at once.

Garnish with a favorite herb after baking.

I keep a bag of mini muffins and sliced baguettes in my freezer for when unexpected guests show up.

Garlicky Shrimp

Cold shrimp and cold shrimp cocktail are typical in the appetizer offerings. Why not kick it up a bit and add a little garlic, Parmesan cheese, and parsley to the mix? This is the type of shrimp cocktail you can serve at any party—and don't serve it with the regular bottled cocktail sauce. A homemade marinara that is served warm sets your Garlicky Shrimp into the applause arena. Expect your platters to be cleared quickly.

makes: 35 shrimp | **preheat:** oven to 400°F
prep time: 10 minutes | **cooking time:** 10 minutes

ingredients

1 lb large raw, tail-on shrimp, cleaned and deveined

2 T extra virgin olive oil

1 lemon, juiced

½ tsp kosher salt

½ tsp black pepper, freshly ground

3 garlic cloves, minced

½ C Parmesan, grated

2 T parsley, chopped

marinara sauce, warmed for dipping (recipe follows)

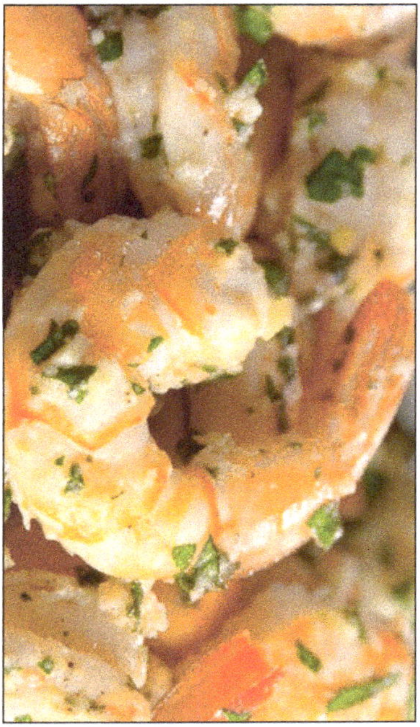

putting it all together

step 1: Preheat oven to 400°F. Line a baking sheet with parchment paper.

step 2: In a large bowl, mix all ingredients, including shrimp.

step 3: Place shrimp on a baking sheet and roast until golden and cooked through, 6-8 minutes. Serve with warm marinara sauce.

Marinara Sauce

makes: 3 cups

ingredients

1 (28-oz) can of whole peeled tomatoes … *if you can get San Marzano tomatoes, grab a can!*

2 T butter

½ white onion, halved

putting it all together

step 1: Place the tomatoes, butter, and the halved onion in a medium saucepan.

step 2: Over medium-high heat, bring to a gentle simmer, then reduce the heat to low. Simmer uncovered for 45 minutes, stirring occasionally and gently crushing the tomatoes with the back of a wooden spoon.

step 2: Remove the saucepan from the heat. Remove onion halves and discard. Season with salt if desired.

Raw or cooked shrimp MUST not sit at room temperature for more than two hours (or one hour if temperatures exceed 90°F / 32°C). Beyond those times,, harmful bacteria multiply rapidly, putting you at a high risk for food poisoning.

For appetizers, it's wise to have an ice bed under cooked shrimp that is to be served cold. For cooked shrimp, it can be stored 3 to 4 days in air tight container in fridge.

Grilled Pesto Shrimp Skewers

Originally, I did this as a main course. Then thinking, why not just for appetizers? With the basil pesto marinade, it's a tad messy, so serve with small plates. I also add forks for those who want to cut the shrimp when it's pulled off the skewer. I've served it many times and have done it with skewers and without. If without, you will roast in the oven.

makes: 8 to 15 full skewers
preheat: Grill or oven at 400°F | **prep time:** 10 minutes
cooking time: 6-8 minutes, until shrimp is pink

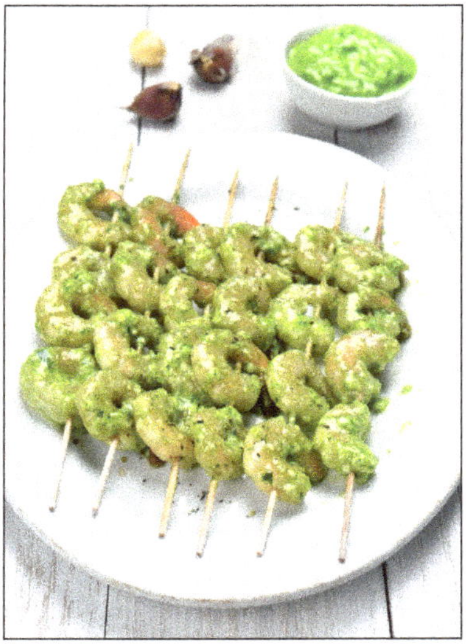

ingredients

1 C fresh basil leaves, chopped

1-2 garlic cloves, minced

¼ C grated Parmigiano Reggiano

2 C basil leaves

½ C olive oil

½ C Parmigiano Reggiano cheese, grated

or

basil pesto sauce from Costco —*add 1 tsp of ground garlic*

1½ lbs jumbo raw shrimp, peeled and deveined

kosher salt and fresh pepper to taste

skewers 4-6 inches, *depending on size of shrimp and length of skewer*

or

skip the skewers … *bake the marinated shrimp and add a toothpick for individual shrimp.*

putting it all together

step 1: Soak wooden skewers in water for at least 30 minutes before adding shrimp onto skewers.

step 2: Make your pesto sauce marinade … combine basil, garlic, Parmesan cheese, salt, and pepper until smooth. Use a food processor to do the pulsing—I have a mini one to do this. Slowly add in the olive oil.

OR, skip and just use the pesto sauce from Costco, eliminating basil, garlic, olive oil, and Parmigiano Reggiano. I add an extra teaspoon of ground garlic.

step 3: Add the shrimp to pesto combo and marinate in a bowl for a few hours.

step 4: Add shrimp to skewers.

step 5: Place the shrimp skewers on the hot grill and cook until pink—flip to other side. Do this with a pan—the marinade will be messy.

step 6: If you skip the skewers, then roast the raw marinated shrimp at 400°F for 5-8 minutes on parchment paper. This goes fast at the cooking stage. Move to your platter and add toothpicks.

Mini Red Lobster Cheddar Biscuits

I've actually brought these when I'm the Appetizer person for one of my foodie groups. When I take on this role, I make 3 different appetizers for multiple nibbling—adding in the biscuits was a surprise! Think of them as an add for soups or just a nibble. Always a hit.

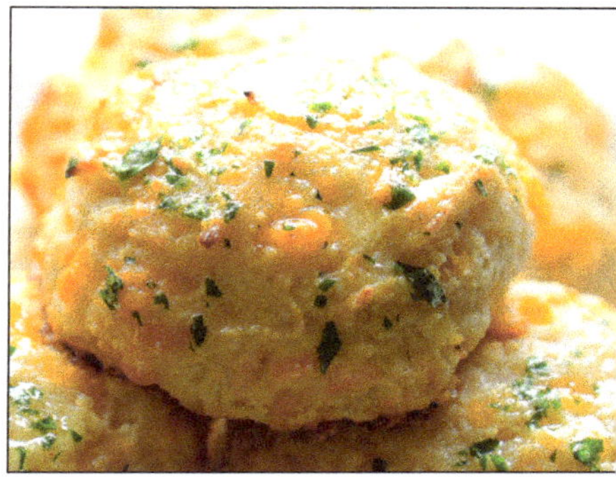

makes: 24 mini biscuits
preheat: oven to 425°F
prep time: 5 to 10 minutes
cooking time: 10–12 minutes

ingredients

Red Lobster®—*you can get the box at Costco, Sam's, your local grocery store, or Amazon. I only use the ORIGINAL mix (allergic to rosemary mix)*

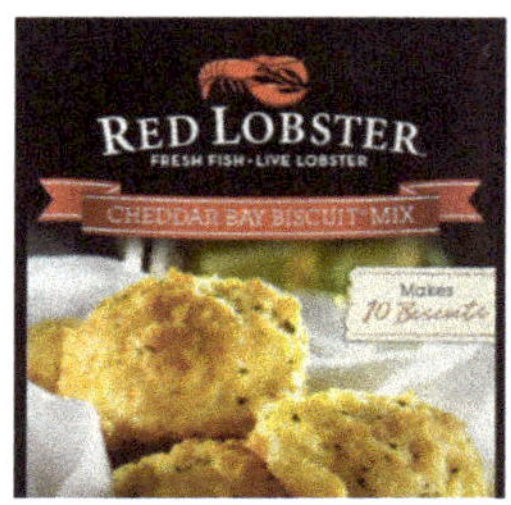

½ to 1 C cheddar cheese, medium or sharp, shredded

½ C butter

Option: ¼ C cilantro, finely chopped *if your guests are not allergic*

putting it all together *My add to it—it's a few steps …*

step 1: Mix the packaged mix with water.

step 2: Add shredded cheddar cheese *(I usually double the cheese).*

step 3: If you add the option of cilantro, finely chop and add in before rolling into mini balls. *Tip:* I will make without the cilantro just in case someone can't eat it. Or, do a half with cilantro, half without.

step 4: Roll into mini balls (no bigger than a walnut) and put on parchment paper … or drop into a greased mini muffin pan.

step 5: Bake for around 10 minutes at 425°F.

step 6: When baking in the oven, melt the butter for the herb mix that comes in the box to drizzle on the baked rolls. I add more butter (at least 50% more) than the box recommends. When ready to do the "drizzle" after biscuits are hot out of the oven, add in the package of herbs and stir. Microwave the butter mix and then spoon it on top of each biscuit.

Serve immediately.

OK ... if you want to do it by SCRATCH ...

here's where I roll up my sleeves and get out the flour!

preheat: oven to 450°F | **prep time:** 15 minutes
cooking time: 10–12 minutes

ingredients

- 2 C all-purpose flour
- 1 T sugar
- 1 T baking powder
- 2 tsp garlic powder
- ½ tsp kosher salt
- ¼ tsp cayenne pepper, optional for a little kick
- 1 C buttermilk
- ½ C unsalted butter, melted
- 1½ C sharp cheddar cheese, shredded

for the topping

- ½ C unsalted butter, melted
- 1 T fresh parsley leaves, chopped
- ½ tsp garlic powder *(more if you love garlic)*

putting it all together

step 1: Preheat oven to 450°F. Line a baking sheet with parchment paper or a silicone baking mat.

step 2: Combine flour, sugar, baking powder, garlic powder, salt and cayenne pepper, if using.

step 3: Whisk together buttermilk and butter. Add to dry ingredients and stir until moist. Gently fold in cheese. *(I do all this with my hands.)*

No buttermilk?—*OK ... here's what you do:*
To 1 C milk, add 1 T of either white vinegar or lemon juice—let sit for 10 minutes.

step 4: Scoop the batter evenly onto the baking sheet (I put parchment paper on mine). Bake for 10-12 minutes, or until golden brown.

step 5: For topping, whisk together butter, parsley and garlic powder in a small bowl. Brush or spoon the tops of the biscuits with the butter mixture.

Serve immediately.

Olive Tapenade with Anchovies

Since I was a kid, I've loved olives ... just about any that I could put in my mouth ... not to mention the open-ended pitted black ones that I could add to each fingertip at Thanksgiving. A tapenade can be a single olive focus or a multi-mixed one. What's a plus for any host is that it comes together in minutes. Better yet, olives beg to be mixed a day or two before you plan on serving them. Use this olive tapenade as either an appetizer or a condiment.

makes: 2 cups | **prep time:** 5 to 10 minutes

ingredients

1 C pitted Kalamata olives, drained, chopped

1 C green olives with pimentos, drained, chopped

1 C Castelvetrano olives, drained, chopped

1 red onion, finely chopped

⅓ C capers

2 T olive oil

2 T lemon juice

2 T fresh basil, chopped

2 anchovy filets, chopped

¼ tsp red pepper flakes

4 oz goat cheese, at least

1 loaf French bread, thinly sliced and toasted **OR** crostini

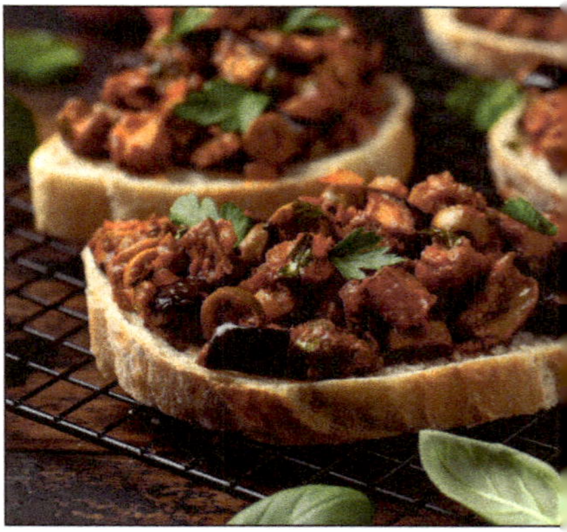

putting it all together

In a bowl, add all the finely chopped olives. Then add capers, red onion, lemon juice, and basil. Stir in olive oil and pepper flakes. Spread goat cheese on the bread or crostini and top with the tapenade. Serve with goat cheese and bread.

Salmon Skewers

Salmon Skewers are a quick, flavorful option for one of your appetizer choices. The marinade you use adds a big flavor. I'm a fan of a honey garlic-based marinade that uses soy sauce, honey, garlic, ginger, and a splash of olive oil. You can do one with herbs that includes olive oil, lemon juice, Dijon mustard, garlic, and dill. Or you can do a cheat and get store-bought to expedite the marinade making. If that's your path, add Kinder's Teriyaki Marinade & Sauce for its garlic-forward flavor or P. F. Chang's Home Menu Teriyaki Sauce—the pineapple add-in is a plus. Another one that I like is the Japanese BBQ Sauce. All can be found in a well-stocked grocery store like Kroger.

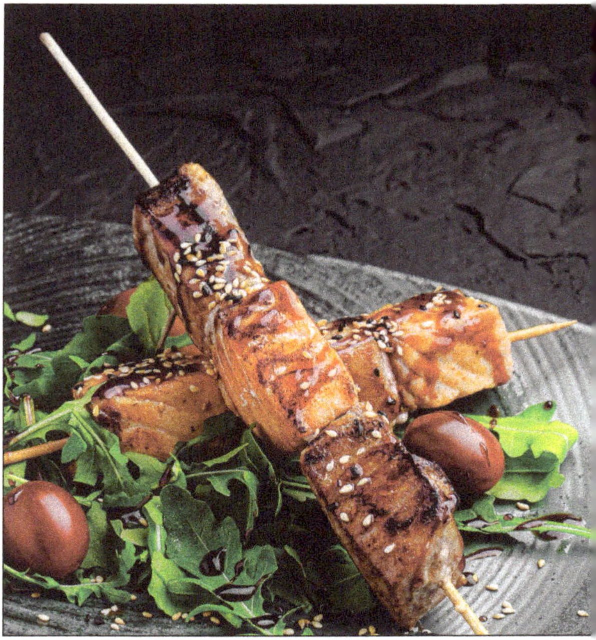

Marinate your salmon for 30 minutes … but no longer than 60 minutes—otherwise it will start turning mushy. Marinate in the refrigerator, and once you remove the salmon, discard the marinade.

Cook it … grilling or broiling works best. Either way is delish and total cook time will be quick—less than 8 minutes. If using wooden skewers, soak them in water for at least 30 minutes to prevent burning and easier removal of the salmon.

makes: 10 to 12 skewers | **prep time:** less than 10 minutes
cooking time: 4-5 minutes each side—top and bottom only

ingredients

4 salmon filets, approximately 6 to 8 oz cut into 1 x 1-½-inch pieces

¼ C olive oil

½ C soy sauce

1 T brown sugar

1 T honey

2 garlic cloves, minced

¾ tsp ginger, ground

sesame seeds—*for sprinkling on baked skewers before serving*

skewers for threading

For the cheat: Have just the salmon filets, sesame seeds, and skewers plus one of the store-bought marinades: Kinder's Teriyaki Marinade & Sauce, P. F. Chang's Home Menu Teriyaki Sauce, or the Japanese BBQ Sauce. Any will work.

putting it all together

step 1: Soak skewers in cold water for at least 30 minutes.

step 2: For a homemade marinade, add all ingredients to a saucepan over medium heat. Bring to a boil for one minute. Your sauce should be thick. If thin, add a slur made of 1 tablespoon cornstarch to 2 tablespoons cold water (never warm or hot). Add into sauce. Stir as it comes to a boil again. Sauce should coat the back of a spoon. Remove from heat—done.

Otherwise, bypass and use one of the store-bought marinades suggested.

step 3: Marinate for 30 minutes.

step 4: Remove salmon from marinade and cut into 1-inch by 1½-inch pieces. Skewer. Sprinkle sesame seeds on before cooking.

step 5: Cook the salmon by grilling, broiling or baking.

step 6 Grilling: Preheat grill to medium-high. Oil your grates and grill for 3-4 minutes per side until the fish is opaque.

step 6 Broiling: Place skewers 6 inches from the heat on a foil-lined baking sheet and broil for 4-5 minutes on two of the sides

Serve immediately.

In the 90s, I spent combined months in Alaska and Canada with my work that involved the books I wrote on conflict resolution for health care professionals. I was mesmerized when I visited a huge fish ladder in Canada. The instinct to travel to fresh water, no matter what, is their final quest.

In Alaska, I spent a day as the voyeur at the river watching huge numbers of salmon ascend a wide river to return to their original places of birth to spawn in fresh water. The majority would die shortly after. At times, they would leap a few feet into the air to clear rocks in the river. And a few bears "fished" packing in unbelievable amounts of fish to fell their bellies.

Being able to enjoy salmon that is freshly caught is a treat. When I'm in Alaska, halibut and salmon are my meals of choice. With a one-day license, I've fished the surrounding seas and returned to land with my catch—sometimes just one, others two or three.

One would be planned for our evening meal. If there were others, they would be taken to the cannery which takes over the cleaning, butchering, and canning under high pressure. Typically canneries operate around the clock. I would ship the finished product home for my family and to share with friends.

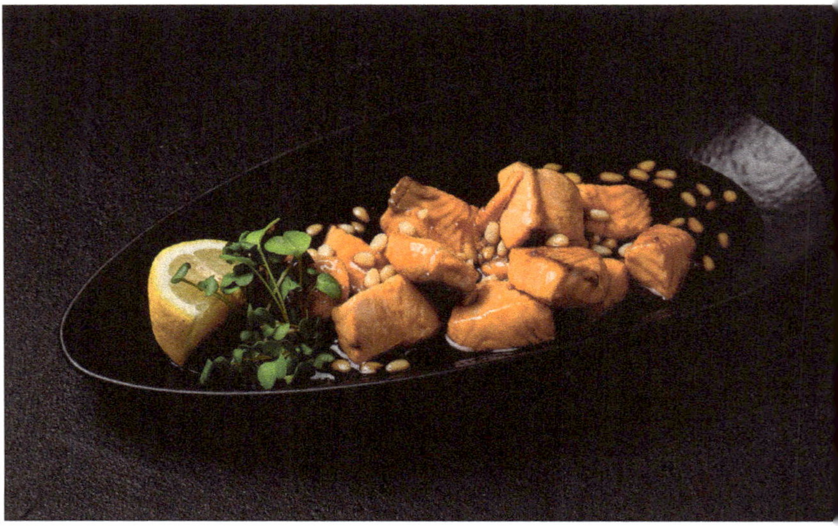

Salmon Teriyaki Bites

Salmon is a welcome addition to appetizers. The prep is so minimal and your guests will think healthy when it's a choice. It pairs well with so many things—cheeses, crackers, and loves a kiss of cream cheese. I love it when it has a marinade in the cooking—and has included a sauce for you to whip up in a few minutes to dribble across the salmon before you place it in the oven.

My adds include artisan crackers, crocks of Boursin, goat cheese, and cream cheese for those who love to pick up with a bread versus just the toothpick bite that is often the norm.

This is one where you can do the sauce ahead, then add to the salmon to bake. I would start the cooking when your guests arrive—social time, drinks, and then serve along with other appetizers you already have available.

makes: 20 to 30 bites | **preheat:** over to 400°F
prep time: 10 minutes | **cooking time:** 12 minutes

ingredient

4 skinless salmon fillets, 2 to 2½ lbs total

ingredients for teriyaki sauce

3 T olive oil

3 T soy sauce

2 T maple syrup—*I use the Costco brand*

2 tsp toasted sesame oil

½ tsp ginger, powder or ground

3 garlic cloves, minced or ¾ tsp ground

¼ tsp crushed red pepper flakes

dill sprigs, small ones

Adds: artisan crackers, crocks of Boursin, goat cheese, and cream cheese for those who love to pick up with a bread or cracker base.

putting teriyaki sauce together

In a small saucepan, combine all ingredients except the salmon. This is a teriyaki sauce with a smidge of a kick from the red pepper flakes. If you don't want the kick, delete. Over medium heat, bring to a boil and immediately drop to a low heat to simmer for less than 2 minutes.

putting it together

step 1: In a baking dish, place the salmon filets with the round flesh side up. Spoon the olive oil and soy sauce mixture evenly over the filets. Move to a preheated over and roast for approximately 14 minutes.

step 2: Once cooked, let the salmon rest a few minutes, then cut into bite-sized pieces. You can arrange them all together with toothpicks. Or, you can add in a favorite cheese—goat, Boursin, or an herbal cream cheese with a side of artisan crackers for those who love to have a base to put the salmon on. Have small pieces of dill to enhance the nibble. I've even included pine nuts that I've pan-roasted to the mix.

seafood

Shrimp, Cucumber, Feta, and Dill Delights

When I want an elegant-looking appetizer that is also easy peasy. The Shrimp, Cucumber, Feta & Dill Delights shout out to me. When you slice the cooked shrimp lengthwise, butterflying them, you get the open, elegant inside curve, which I love to see. Or you can leave them whole. You can put both halves on your cracker or baguette slice, or just one. The result is an inviting eye candy for your guests. Adding the easy crunch of a few English cucumber slices and a sprig of dill bookended with a creamy cheese spread, you get a salty feta creation and a happy dance for your guests.

This appetizer is an easy-peasy one that takes minimal time to put together.

makes: 12 to 15 Delights | **prep time:** 25 minutes
cooking time: No cooking with precooked shrimp. If baking baguette slices, 10 – 12 minutes at 350°F

ingredients

12-24 medium to large shrimp, tails off, already cooked—*If you want to kickup the quality of shrimp, get the raw wild red Argentina shrimp—mine come from Costso.*

1 English cucumber, sliced

crackers or cocktail breads for spreading *(I like pumpernickel or rye)* or baguette slices—both plain and lightly toasted

½ lb feta – *if you can get European, get it*—French, Greek, or Bulgarian, otherwise American slab

½ C dry white wine

1 tsp kosher salt for cucumbers—*if cooking raw shrimp, an additional 1 tsp kosher salt to water*

½ tsp garlic salt

putting it all together

step 1: Thaw pre-cooked shrimp. If cooking raw, add wine and kosher salt to water and cook until shrimp turns opaque, pearly pink in color, and is firm. Its shape is similar to a loose letter "C."

step 2: Marinate shrimp in wine and garlic salt for 15 minutes. Remove and butterfly them.

step 3: Peel a seedless English cucumber. Slice into ⅛- or ¼-inch slices and drain for 15 minutes in a colander. I add salt to help the draining.

step 4: Crackers-your choice, cocktail breads-your choice, or baguette slices ¼- or ⅜-inch thick. Bake baguette slices brushed with olive oil and a sprinkle of garlic salt.

step 5: Spread feta on baguette, cocktail bread, or crackers. Layer two slices of cucumber. Add shrimp and top with a small sprig of dill.

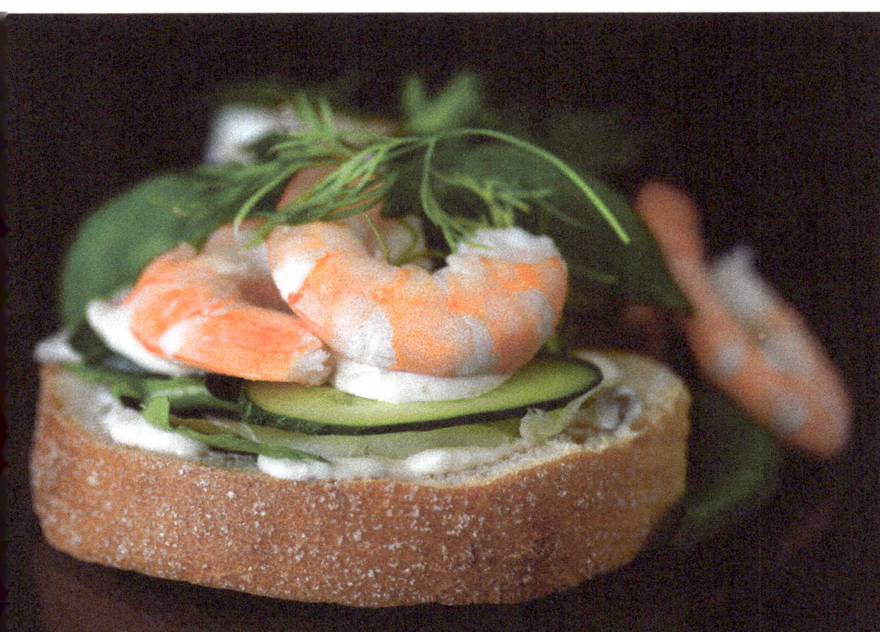

Shrimp Cucumber Open Bites

I'm all for a variety of food items. I've done gatherings with over a dozen appetizers to choose from … most of my friends feel that by the time they leave, they've had dinner … but it's all in a variety of bites.

My Shrimp Cucumber Open Bites became one of those fillers. Starting with cocktail bread squares or slices from a baguette, with the first layer a cream cheese, then they are piled with a few thin slices of cucumber, a tomato slice, a shrimp, and a wee bit of fresh dill. Don't be surprised if your guests want two.

makes: 15 Bites

prep time: 20 minutes | **cooking time:** No cooking

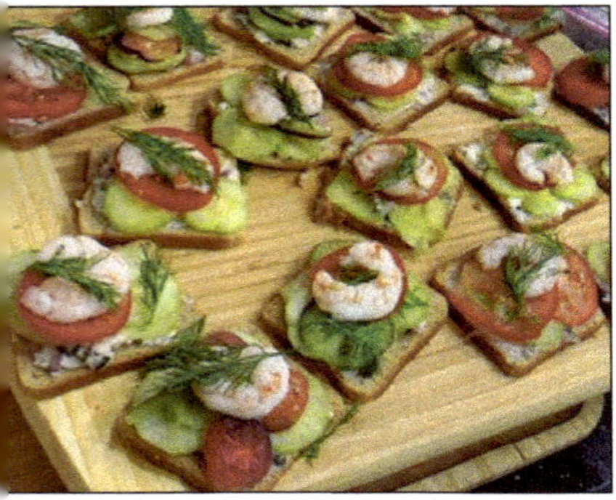

ingredients

1 lb shrimp, medium or large size, cooked and butterflied

6-8 Roma tomatoes, sliced thin

1-2 English cucumbers, peeled and sliced thin

cocktail breads—*I like rye and pumpernickel*

2 different cream cheese spreads—Philadelphia herb, onion, or garlic

dill, fresh

putting it all together

step 1: Cook or get precooked shrimp—butterfly them by slitting in half lengthwise. them. You will use half a shrimp on each open-faced bread.

step 2: Starting with cocktail bread squares or baguette slices, generously layer the first layer a cream cheese. Then add a few thin slices of cucumber, a tomato slice, a shrimp, and a wee bit of fresh dill on top.

Sometimes I squeeze a few drops of lemon on the shrimp and

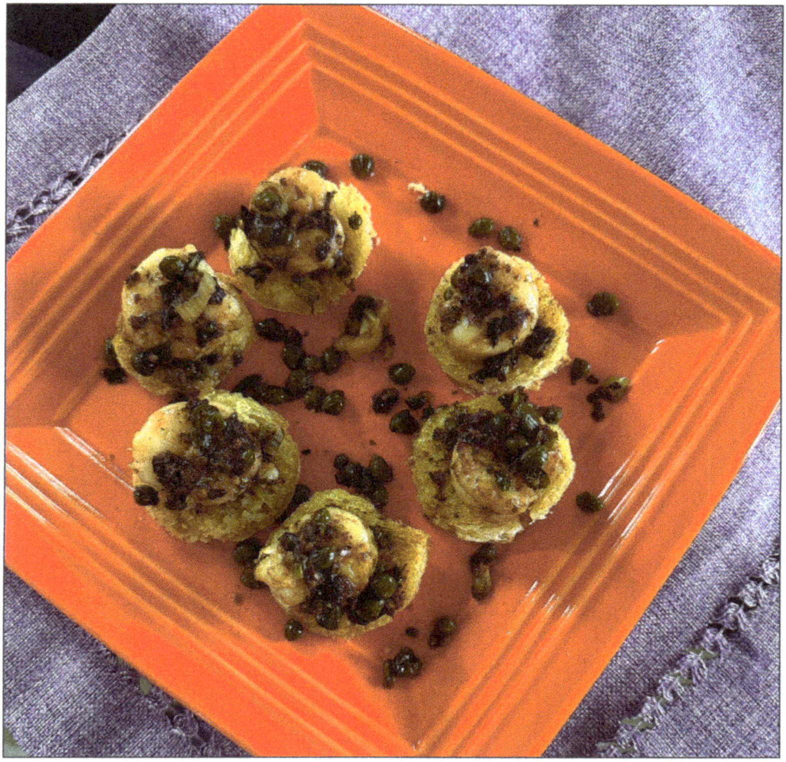

Shrimp Scampi Toasties

I've always loved shrimp scampi. The simplicity of the shrimp combined with butter, garlic, and lemon was on my perfect dinner list. Sometimes with angel hair pasta and a salad. Voilá dinner is complete. Why not slip it into the appetizer arena without the pasta and add toasted sourdough bread to the mix for a base? Why not indeed!

Visiting my local farmer's market, I found the perfect fresh sourdough bread in half inch slices. As I looked at it, my thoughts bubbled—why not cut circles in the bread and make a toastie base for something? Back in my kitchen, a small glass was turned upside down to cut into the bread. Next, I toasted them lightly in the oven. Next was prepping the shrimp and getting my ingredients gathered to make the scampi sauces are in. These Toasties are in the easy peasy.

Cooking the shrimp, then the sauce, I stacked all on top of the toasted round and drizzled with the lemon sauce on top. A mouth sensation was created. When I did my first sample, the platter became our meal—I thought my husband was going to lick the plate I served them on!

You now have sautéed shrimp in a delicious garlic butter to soak with a toastie base to soak up all the flavors. And there's a bonus … the aromas in your kitchen are divine—it's the butter, garlic, and lemon that sets the stage.

makes: 15 to 20 Toasties | **preheat:** oven to 350°F
prep time: 7 minutes | **cooking time:** 15 minutes

ingredients

1 pound raw, deveined shrimp … about 15 per pound. Remove tails.

1 sourdough bread loaf, thickly sliced or whole

2 lemons, juiced

4 T extra virgin olive oil, divided

3 garlic cloves, peeled and minced

½ C capers

½ C dry white wine

3 T fresh lemon juice

¼ C scallions, thinly sliced

6 T unsalted butter

¾ tsp sea salt

7 grates of freshly cracked black pepper

ingredient for scampi sauce

2 T fresh parsley leaves, lightly chopped (for garnish)

putting it all together

step 1: Clean and devein shrimp and remove tails.

step 2: To marinate shrimp: combine 2 garlic cloves-minced, 1 T olive oil. Cover in bowl or place shrimp in a sealed bag. Set aside and refrigerate 25 minutes.

step 3: Make half inch slices from whole loaf or lay out already sliced bread. Make rounds (or squares) with a cookie cutter or the rim of a small glass pushed into the bread. Place the bread toastie on baking tray in a preheated 350 degree oven and toast for 5 minutes until lightly golden around the edges. Not crisp, just lightly golden. Set aside.

step 4: In a skillet, add 1 tablespoon of olive oil at medium heat. Add the marinated shrimp. Do not stir them. Lightly brown on first side, then cook for one minute. Turn the shrimp over, lightly brown second side. Cook for one minute. Shrimp is cooked. Remove to a plate. Keep any bits from shrimp in the pan.

step 5: Add 2 tablespoons of olive oil to pan at low-medium heat. Add minced garlic. Stir one minute with any bits. Add white wine and lemon juice to make your lemon sauce. Add scallions. Bring to a boil, stirring another minute, until slightly reduced.

step 6: Reduce heat on stove. Add butter, 2 tablespoons at a time—swirl in, using a fork. Continue with the rest of the butter until the sauce has emulsified. Stir capers and sea salt.

step 7: Stack with a toastie at base, then shrimp, then garlic lemon sauce with capers.

Serve either on a platter where guests serve themselves or place 2 toasties on a small individual plates. I would include small forks. You may want to make extra toasties to add in a bowl so that they can be used to soak up the sauce.

seafood

Smoked Salmon Super Dip

Dips are always an add to most soirees. As I put this together, my garden pots were full of fresh dill. I usually have frozen salmon filets stashed in the freezer and cream cheese and Greek yogurt in the fridge. Hmmm … a creamy dip, with a kick of horseradish was talking to me.

If you are a bagel fan, why not turn your dip to a spread? And a plus, you can make this the day before you plan to serve it.

makes: 2 cups | **prep time:** 10 minutes | **cooking time:** none

ingredients

½ lb. smoked salmon, finely chopped

¾ C Greek yogurt

8 oz cream cheese, softened

1 T horseradish

3 T dill

2 T capers

1 T lemon juice

2 tsp lemon zest

Salt and pepper

putting it all together

step 1: Combine the cream cheese, Greek yogurt, horseradish, lemon juice, and lemon zest in a food processor. Pulse until smooth—this dip should be extra creamy and spreadable.

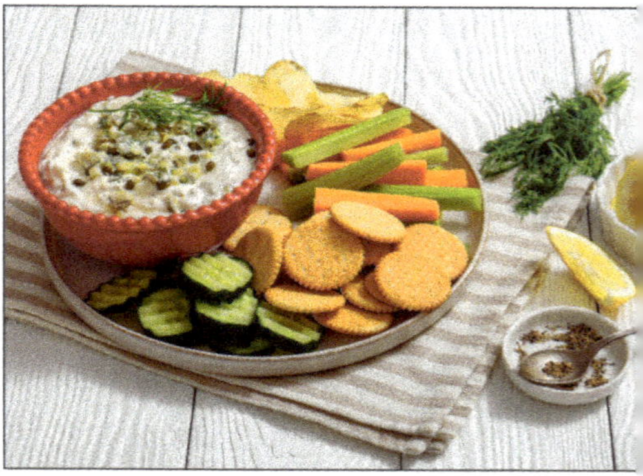

step 2: Gently fold smoked salmon, capers, and dill. Season with salt and pepper to taste. Refrigerate.

step 3: Serve with crackers and crudités. There's always the usual: celery, carrots, and zucchini. Stretch—add red and yellow pepper strips, snow peas, asparagus spears, cornlettes, green beans … *what else?*

Stuffed Mushrooms with Crab and Cheese

Welcome to the mushroom world. Baked mushrooms and crab are always a go-to in my home for seafood lovers at my gatherings. I use large button mushrooms or baby bella ones with stems removed and lump crab as the filling. Why? They are firm, perfect for baking with a filling. Mushroom caps are the perfect filling vessel for so many goodies—crab is one of my favorites.

Either mushroom is of the same species. The only difference is age. Button mushrooms are harvested young and milder in flavor. Baby bellas mature longer developing their brownish color, giving you a richer, earthier, and meatier mushroom.

I use them both.

makes: 20 to 25 mushrooms | **preheat:** oven to 375°F
prep time: 10 minutes | **cooking time**: 16-18 minutes

ingredients

20-25 mushrooms—*your choice of mushrooms*

8-12 oz lump crab meat

½ C mixed cheddar cheeses, shredded

½ C freshly grated Parmesan, plus more for topping

4 oz cream cheese

4 scallions (green onions), thinly sliced

2 garlic cloves, minced

½ C panko

1 lemon, juiced

1 tsp each salt and black pepper

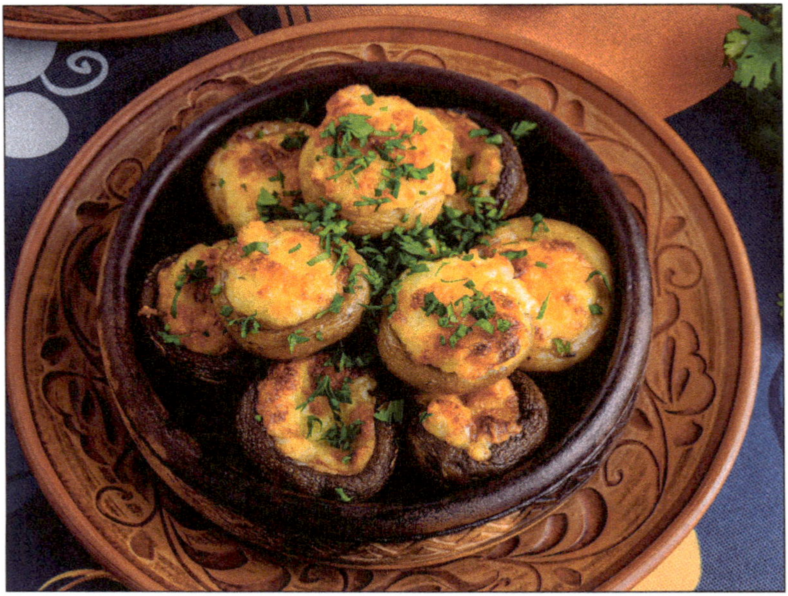

putting it all together

step 1: Clean the outside of the mushrooms with a damp paper towel and remove the stems. Reserve stems for another purpose or toss. If there is any moisture inside the cap, gently dab the inside of each mushroom with the paper towel to soak up excess moisture.

step 2: In a large bowl, mix all ingredients except the mushrooms. OK, I mix with my hands to make sure the cheeses are really mixed in.

step 3: Fill each mushroom with a heaping teaspoon of the crab meat mixture and place on an ungreased, shallow baking dish or cookie sheet. Dust the top of the mushrooms with more grated Parmesan and bake until the tops of the mushrooms are golden brown.

step 4: Remove from oven, and gently squeeze a few drops of lemon juice on top of each and serve immediately.

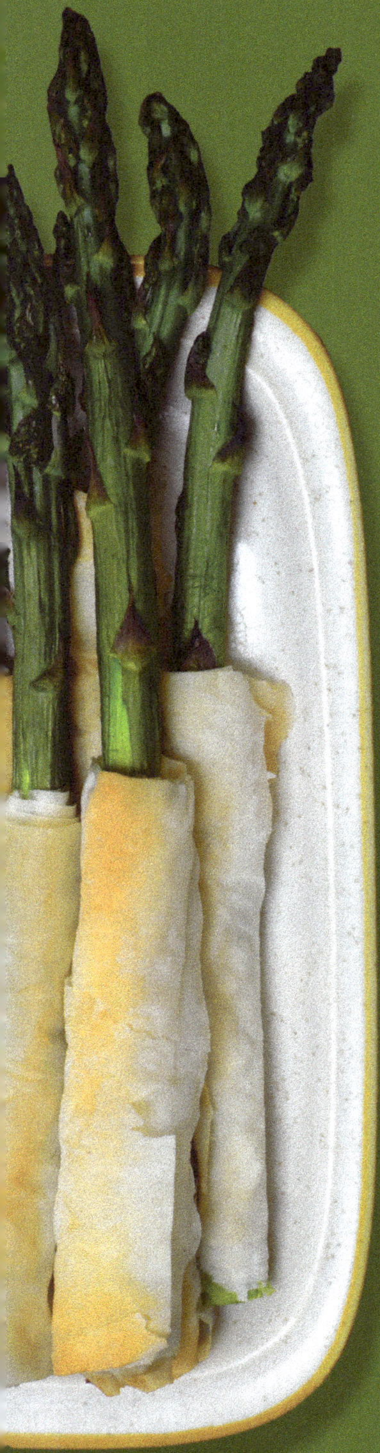

veggies

Artichoke Hearts with a Kiss of Paprika

Prep and cooking time is less than 20 minutes. Makes 6 to 12, depending on how many artichokes are in a jar. A 12 oz jar usually has 6 to 12 artichokes, depending on size. I plan on two per person.

I love it when I can use a favorite veggie—artichokes are one. Whether whole and dipping in a bit of mayo or added to a salad, it's always fun to discover quick, easy ways to add to an appetizer array. Why not artichokes?

These start with jars of drained marinated artichoke hearts and dipping them into a beer batter for frying. Add a little salt and it's a TaDah! I promise they will disappear quickly when your friends discover them.

makes: 12 to 20 Hearts | **prep time:** 10 minutes
cooking time: 20 minutes; cook in small batches for 2–3 minutes each batch

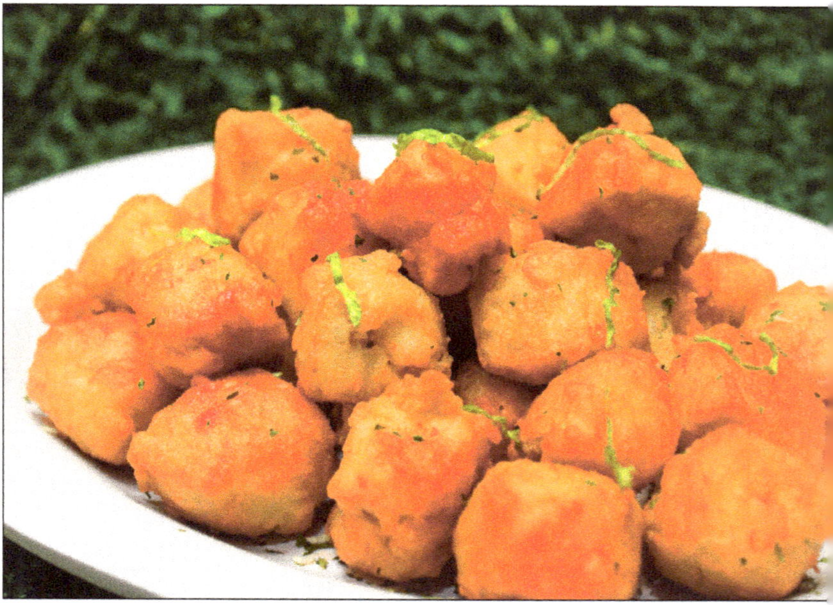

ingredients

2 jars of artichokes

1 C flour—*add more flour if needed for thickening*

¾ C beer

olive oil or avocado oil for frying

smoked paprika—*you will sprinkle on top when cooked*

sea salt—*you will sprinkle on top when cooked*

putting it all together

step 1: Drain the artichokes—whatever marinade lingers—keep it … it will add to each bite. Whisk the flour into the beer. Dip each artichoke into the batter, coating evenly.

step 3: In a pan, heat approximately 1 inch of oil to medium/high and drop in your battered artichoke until golden—about a minute. If you use less oil, you are turning two times quickly. Drain on paper towel. Cook in small batches of six.

step 4: Immediately sprinkle with paprika and sea salt. *Definitely serve warm with a cool beverage … beer?*

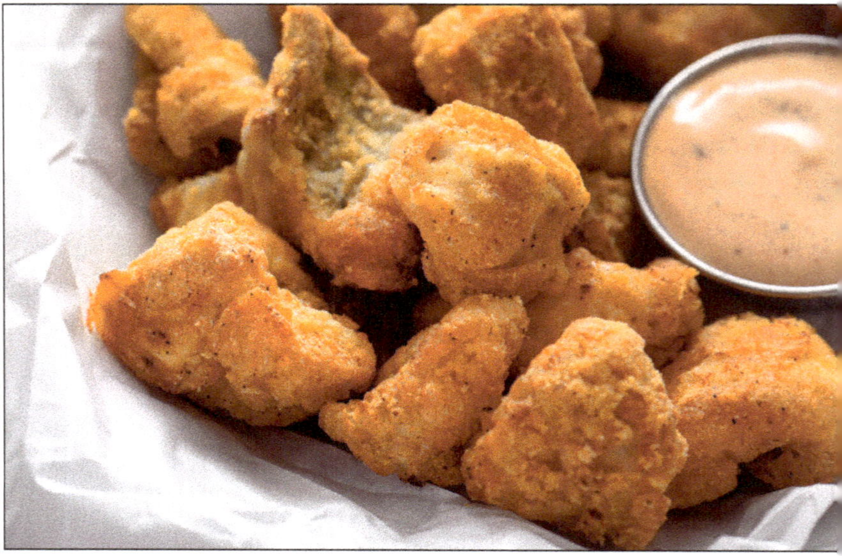

Artichoke Hearts with Sauces

I always welcome the summer months when artichokes are in full bloom. Living in Northern California for over 20 years, the Castroville Artichoke Festival was a favorite destination in North Monterey County. These appetizers are a crowd favorite.

Baked artichoke appetizers are often paired with rich and creamy sauces or tangy dips to complement each bite. Think **Lemon-Garlic Aioli** *(recipes follows), warm drawn butter,* **Honey Mustard with a Kiss of Raspberries** *(recipes follows), or a* **Creamy Pesto** *(recipes follows). Ooh … my mouth waters as I write this.*

makes: 12 to 20 artichokes, depending on how many in a can/jar
preheat: oven to 400°F | **prep time:** 20 minutes
cooking time: 17 minutes

ingredients

- 2 cans/jars artichoke hearts
- 1 tsp garlic powder
- 1 C grated Parmesan cheese
- 1 C plain breadcrumbs
- ½ C butter, melted

putting it all together

step 1: Line a baking sheet with parchment paper. Set aside.

step 2: Drain artichoke hearts, put in a bowl, and pat dry with paper towel.

step 3: In a small bowl, combine melted butter and garlic powder.

step 4: In another small bowl, combine Parmesan cheese and breadcrumbs.

step 5: Dip each artichoke heart quarter in butter first, then breadcrumbs. Place on prepared baking sheet. Repeat with all artichokes.

step 6: Bake artichokes for 17 minutes or until golden brown. Turn once halfway through baking.

step 7: Let cool to room temperature. Place on a serving dish. Add a sauce …

Lemon-Garlic Aioli

Get ready to whip up a quick and creamy lemon garlic aioli using five ingredients—salt and pepper are two of them. It's a sauce that is punchy and perfect for dipping—pita chips, crostini, fries, even a spread on sandwiches that welcome a lemon tang.

makes: ¾ cup | **prepping and chilling time:** 20 minutes

ingredients

¾ C mayonnaise

2–3 garlic cloves, minced

1– 2 T lemon juice

1 tsp lemon zest

½ tsp each of kosher salt and freshly cracked black pepper

putting it all together

step 1: Combine the minced garlic, lemon juice, and lemon zest. Let it sit for 5-10 minutes to allow the garlic flavor to mellow and blend with the citrus. Add the mayonnaise to the bowl.

step 2: Whisk everything together until the mixture is completely smooth and creamy. Add salt and pepper to taste. If you prefer a brighter, tangier sauce, stir in an extra splash of lemon juice.

step 3: Cover and refrigerate for at least 15-20 minutes before serving.

Creamy Basil Pesto

Herby, cheesy, garlicky pesto is a perfect sauce to have around, and adding one extra ingredient takes it in a different direction. And that's fresh cream to make it a creamy pesto sauce, perfect for dipping pita chips, naked crostini, and just about anything you can scoop away with.

I could have you mash a few bunches of basil, adding in olive oil, Parmesan cheese, lots of garlic, and the ingredients to create the true homemade version. My favorite: Costco Kirkland Basil Pesto is outstanding. Do the shortcut—get it, then dry roast pecans, pine nuts, or walnuts as your add.

makes: 1½ cups | **prepping and chilling time:** 25 minutes

ingredients

1 C Costco basil pesto

½ C heavy cream, coconut cream for nondairy options

⅓ C raw pine nuts or walnuts—*do a dry roast in a skillet for a few minutes, then chop for sprinkling on top*

½–¾ C Parmesan cheese

basil leaves for garnish

putting it all together

step 1: Dry roast nuts for a few minutes in a skillet on the stove top.

step 1: Combine pesto with Parmesan. Stir in cream. If need thinner, add more cream. Done.

step 1: Refrigerate until ready to use. *Sprinkle nuts on top … add a few basil leaves for eye candy.*

Honey Mustard with a Kiss of Raspberries

makes: ¾ cup | **prepping and chilling time:** 20 minutes

ingredients

½ C mayonnaise

3 T Dijon mustard

2 T honey

1 T lemon juice

3 T raspberry jam, seedless

putting it all together

Combine all and whisk away. Refrigerate at least 15-20 minutes to let the magic blending happen.

Asparagus Phyllo Pipes

In the past, asparagus was a spring-to-summer veggie. Now you can get your hands on them year-round. I've had so many appetizers where either the asparagus is withered or almost tasteless when pastry dough is used—it takes too long to do the baking and zaps the asparagus. Using phyllo dough drops the oven time, and the asparagus has a chance to still be asparagus. The **Lemon Dill Sauce** *(recipe follows) is an accompaniment.*

makes: 24 pipes | **preheat:** oven to 375°
prep time: 35 minutes | **cooking time:** 16–20 minutes

ingredients

24 asparagus spears, trimmed to 4 or 5 inches

4 sheets of phyllo pastry dough

2 Boursin packages—*or use another herb soft cheese*

3 T butter, melted

salt for precooking asparagus

putting it all together

step 1: Preheat oven and bring a pan of salted water to a boil. Have a bowl of ice-cold water ready close by.

step 2: Quickly dropped asparagus into the boiling pan for no more that 90 seconds. Remove at once and drop into ice-cold water bath to stop the heat. Drain the bowl and place asparagus on paper towels. Dry.

step 3: Roll out your phyllo and cut each sheet into 24 rectangles. On the short edge of each sheet, place a dry asparagus with the spear head poking out.

step 4: Cut the Boursin into 24 pieces. They will soften quickly. Reshape to match most of the asparagus stem. Position the cheese portion in the middle next to the spear.

step 5: With the melted butter, brush the phyllo around the spear and cheese. Now roll it so the spear and cheese are compact within the phyllo. If you do this too tight, the phyllo will split in the final bake. Brush more butter on the rolled phyllo pipe to seal.

step 6: Place on parchment papered baking sheet with the seal side down. Bake until golden, approximately 15 minutes. Cool on rack and serve either as a single appetizer or add **Lemon Dill Sauce** (recipe follows).

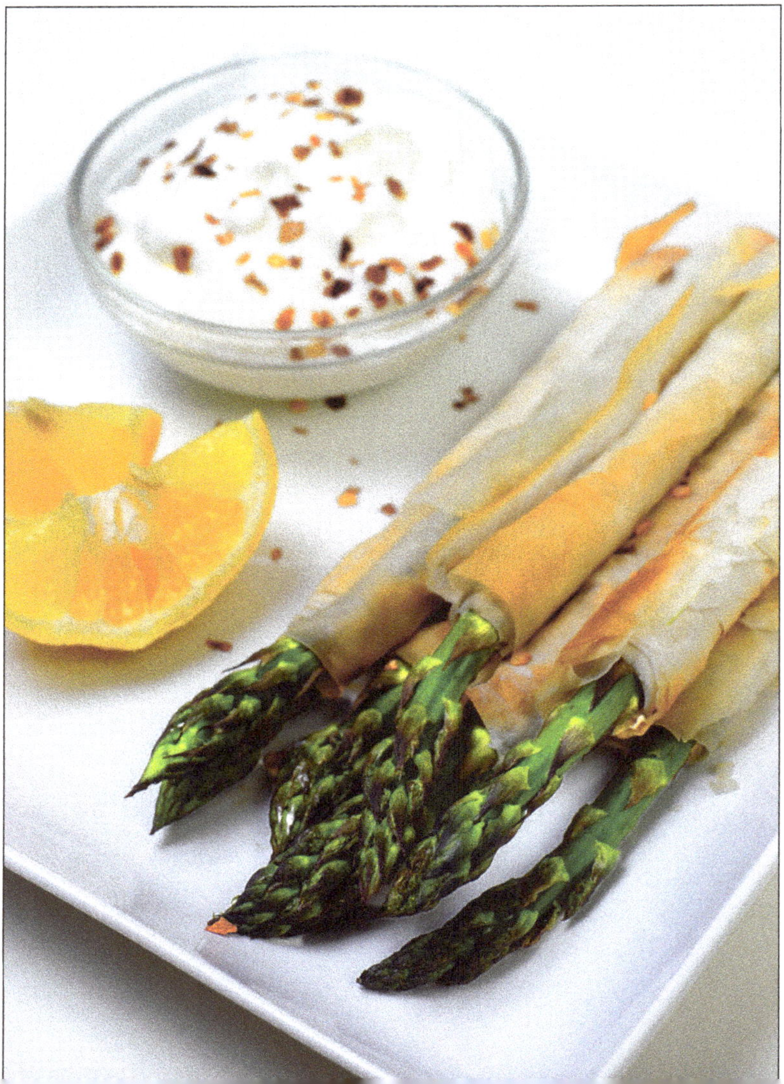

Lemon Dill Sauce

Lemon butter dill sauce can easily be used for enhancing a dish, like chicken or fish … or a vegetable. Why not the Asparagus Phyllo Pipes for a dip? Made with a dry white wine and fresh dill, it's only ten minutes in the making. Basil is also a good substitute for the dill.

makes: 2 cups
prep time: 3 minutes | **cooking time:** 10 minutes

ingredients

1½ C dry white wine

4 T shallots, minced

6 T lemon juice

2 sticks (or 1 cup) butter, cut into 12 pieces

2 T dill, chopped

salt and pepper to taste

putting it all together

step 1: Combine white wine, shallots, and lemon juice in a small saucepan and boil over high heat until reduced to 1 cup, about 6 minutes.

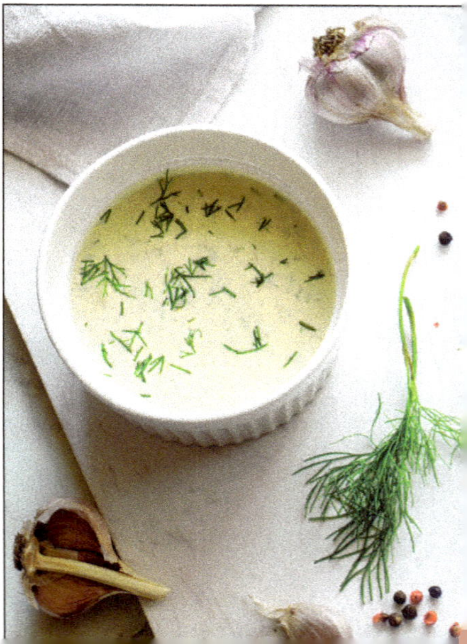

step 2: Reduce heat to low and add butter, one piece at a time, whisking until melted before adding more.

step 3: Remove pan from heat. Stir in fresh dill.

Season to taste with salt and pepper.

Bocconcini Spikes aka Mozzarella Spikes

Every host wants something a bit different and takes basically no time to put together. Spikes need only a few ingredients—like five! You will need short skewers to hold each together. Bocconcini cheese comes from buffalo milk.Mozzarella is often substituted for it.

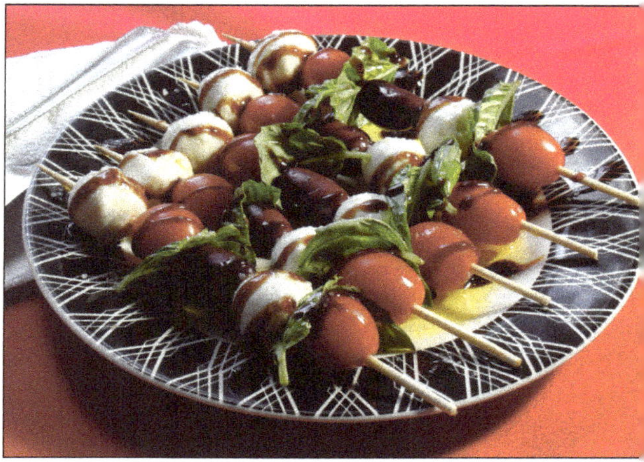

makes: about 20 spikes
prep time: 30 minutes
cooking time: none

ingredients

40 mozzarella mini balls

basil leaves—*these will be your "wrappers"*

40 cherry tomatoes

20 Kalamata olives, whole pitted

balsamic vinegar

olive oil

skewers, 4 to 6 inches long

putting it all together

You can start with a basil leaf on your skewer or use one or two as a weaver between the mozzarella ball, small tomato, then a Kalamata olive onto the skewer-best in the middle. Do with all and create your platter. If you like a bit of balsamic vinegar and olive oil, sprinkle a little when skewers are on the platter. Done.

Fast Cream Cheese Sweet Pepper Bites

When I first discovered sweet mini peppers, they called out to me. It was love at first sight … and eventually bite. The yellow and red are my favorites. Add a creamy filling. They are an ideal no-brainer to add to your nibble mix. For the cream cheese, you can use plain, or enhance your flavoring with one of the herb/condiment variety in the dairy and refrigerated products section of your grocery store.

I love the variety—simple cream cheese, a kick up to a mix of some sort, or maybe a twist with a goat cheese or feta, which begs me to add in basil or dill. I've played with a Mediterranean theme mixing one of the creamy European fetas, Kalamata olives, finely chopped tomatoes and a sprinkling of basil. Don't forget a few capers. Use your imagination.

Years ago, I found a set of grapefruit spoons. With the serrated edging, it's a "tool" I use so often that a few of them are included in a standing container by my stove that contain all odds and ends of spoons. I use spoons for tasting throughout a cooking session. The grapefruit spoons are perfect for scooping out the seeds and ribs of the peppers.

makes: 12-15 pepper bites
prep time: 10 minutes | **cooking time:** none

ingredients

1 package of mini peppers—*I get from Costco*

12 oz cream cheese or your substitute, softened

¾ C sharp cheddar cheese, shredded—*Feta and goat cheese can be added or substituted.*

¼ tsp garlic powder

¼ tsp onion powder

1 T chives, finely chopped

balsamic vinegar

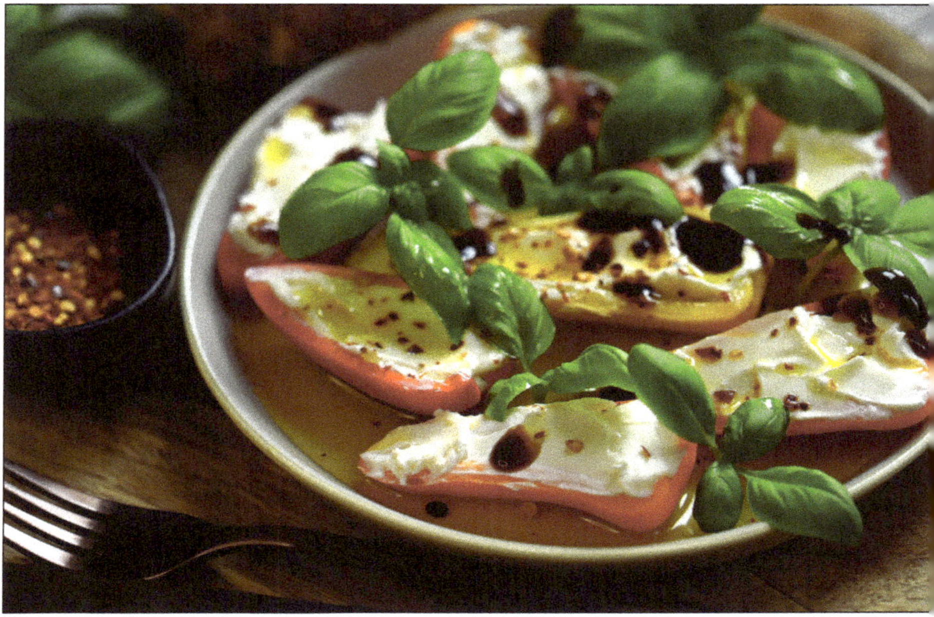

putting it all together

step 1: Wash and dry the mini peppers. Cut in half lengthwise. Remove the seeds and ribs.

step 2: Soften cream cheese and mix in shredded cheddar, feta or goat, garlic powder, and onion powder in a bowl. Stir until smooth.

step 3: Fill each pepper half with your cheese mixture.

Garnishes? Why not … add a sprinkling of chives. Or basil. Maybe a drizzle of balsamic vinegar. If you are a fan of Everything But The Bagel, a few pinches on top of each adds a little more eye pop and taste. Since I'm a fan of capers, I sometimes add them, too.

Serve immediately.

Garlic Butter Mushroom Bites

Mushrooms are one of the most versatile vegetables. They offer earthy, rich, and savory flavors that work well as bite-sized appetizers.

An excellent side dish for sit-down dinners—casual for dress-up gatherings. An add to salads. A welcome addition to soups and stews. And definitely a stand-alone appetizer. That's where my Garlic Butter Mushroom Bites come in. Mushrooms go with so many things. And the best part: so simple to put together.

makes: 20 to 25 Bites | **preheat:** oven to 425°F
prep time: 10 minutes | **cooking time:** 20 minutes

ingredients

1 lb or 20-25 Cremini mushrooms, big ones halved

3 T melted butter

1 T balsamic vinegar

3 minced garlic cloves or 1½ tsp garlic powder

salt, pepper to taste

2 tsp dried parsley or fresh parsley, chopped

toothpicks

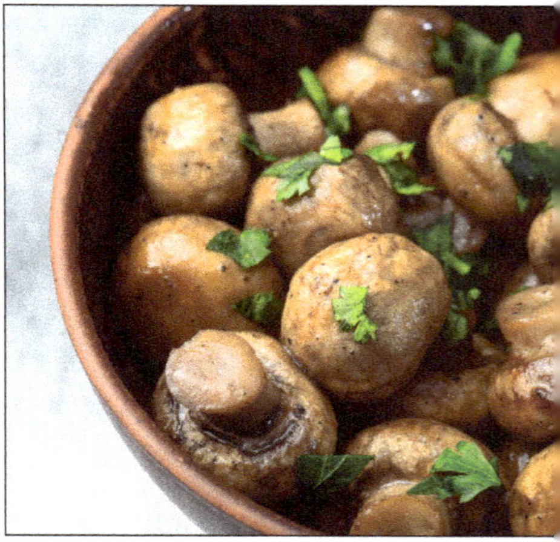

putting it all together

step 1: Clean mushrooms and halve them if large. Trim stems.

step 2: Toss mushrooms in a bowl with melted butter, balsamic, garlic, salt, and pepper.

step 3: Spread evenly on a baking sheet and roast at 425°F until tender and browned. Garnish with fresh chopped parsley.

Use toothpicks for serving.

Mini Stuffed Sweet Peppers

This is where an "anything goes" and "whatever" attitude works. Mini stuffed peppers are excellent adds to any appetizer assortment. The minis are easily picked up to deliver a few tasty bites to whatever you fill them with. If served raw, there's a crunch to them which I love. If stuff and bake, your guests may say, "I never thought of doing that."

You can serve them cold, which is the most common for a finger food appetizer, usually with a cream cheese … or baked so there is a goo factor and warmth. Hmm, adding a taco mix to them would surprise your guests—hello Cinco de Mayo—or bringing a Mediterranean flavor with sliced Kalamata olives, finely chopped tomatoes and a kiss of basil or pesto.

From a no-brainer cream cheese to a more intricate and hearty add. Sometimes it's what I have in the refrigerator when I open it that becomes the add. Without giving a full recipe, this one is to generate ideas for fills.

Your filling will be in the heaping tablespoon range for most of your peppers. Adjust, depending upon the pepper half size.

makes: as many sweet peppers you stuff | **preheat:** oven to 400°F
prep time: 10 minutes | **cooking time:** 12-15 minutes, served cold

ingredients

1 small bag mini sweet peppers

cheeses: cream, Monterey jack, pepper jack, mozzarella, bleu or gorgonzola, goat, feta, Parmesan—*the best cheese choice ultimately comes down to your preferred flavors and types.*

adds: chopped olives, tomatoes, dill, basil, bacon bits, salsa, taco seasoning, balsamic glaze, *what else?*

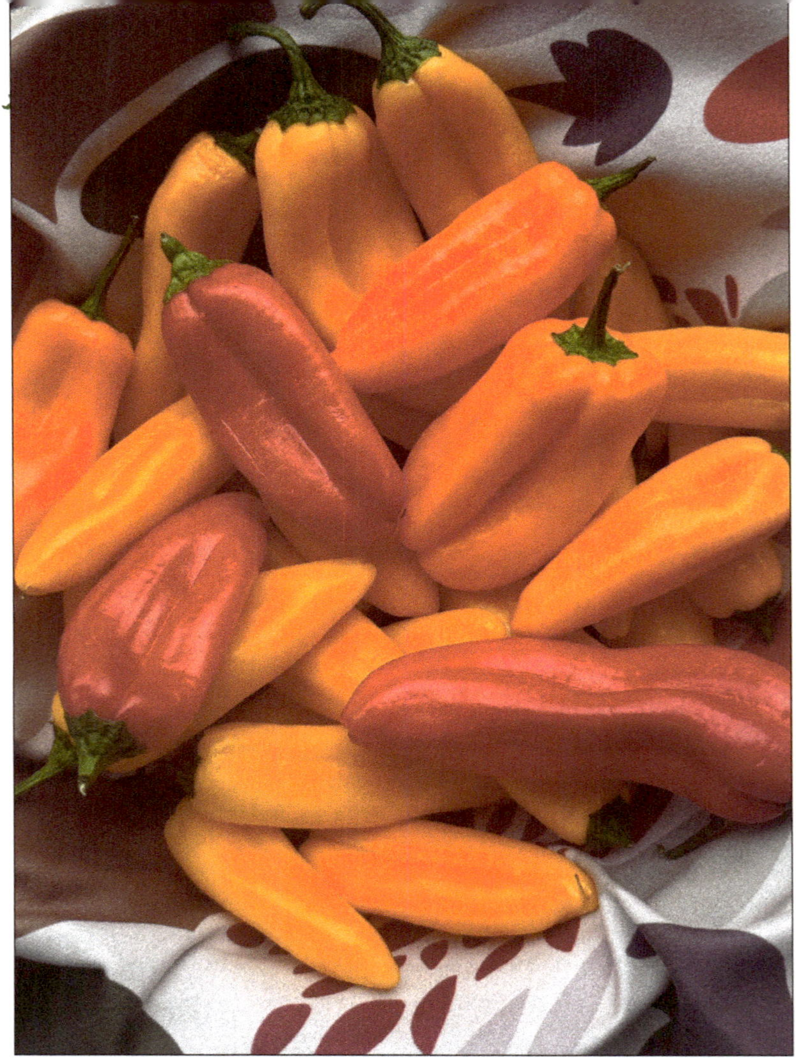

For Creamy/Tangy Taste Sensation

Cream Cheese & Goat Cheese: When you stuff your peppers, a soft cheese base works best. Mixing cream cheese with feta or herbs creates an easy spreadable filling.

For Smooth Melt & Mild Flavor

Mozzarella: It melts beautifully into a gooey, stretchy layer without overpowering the flavor of anything else you add to the pepper.

Monterey Jack: Pairs well with almost any additional fillings.

For Bold, Savory Kick

Sharp Cheddar: Adds a rich, tangy flavor that pairs well if you add meat or rice to the pepper.

Pepper Jack: If you want a little heat, this is your best option. It's Monterey Jack infused with jalapeños.

Cream Cheese based ... cold or baked

Bacon & Cheddar: Softened cream cheese mixed with shredded cheddar, green onions, and crispy cooked and crumbled bacon.

Herb & Garlic: Cream cheese or Boursin blended with garlic powder, dill, chives, and a squeeze of lemon juice. Top with Everything Bagel Seasoning.

Goat Cheese & Parmesan: A mixture of soft goat cheese, Parmesan, minced garlic, sea salt, and fresh cracked pepper.

Mediterranean: Feta mashed with cream cheese, topped with sliced olives (green and Kalamata), diced tomatoes, and fresh basil.

putting it all together

step 1: It always starts with the prep. Cut the mini sweet peppers in half lengthwise. If there is a stem, leave it on one of the sides for a built-in handle. Scoop out any seeds and membranes. There should be very few.

step 2: If serving cold, assemble your filling. Fill half pepper with about one tablespoon of filling. When done, refrigerate if not serving right away.

If serving hot, stay close to the oven. Assemble your mix, fill pepper and place it in a baking dish for roasting at 400°F for 12-15 minutes. You want the peppers to be tender. You want the cheese to be hot, melted, and slightly bubbling. If it's a veggie mix, the degree of

Mushroom Nibbles with Dipping Sauce

If you like mushrooms, hopefully your guests do too. This is a whole mushroom buried within a delicious batter and dipped into a sauce of choice. You may have discovered a tasty treat that is uncomplicated to make.

Both fried and baked mushrooms can be yummy, yet they can have a different audience. If the eater likes crispy or a deep-fried crunch that is juicy, there's a spot to indulge the sensation. More cleanup is required, and frying odors may linger. If you want to enjoy mushrooms without the deep-frying process, baking them is the healthy, less messy alternative. Of course, the crunch isn't there, but the taste is!

makes: 14 Nibbles | **prep time:** 20 minutes
cooking time: 5 minutes per fried mushroom batch; 20 minutes for baking

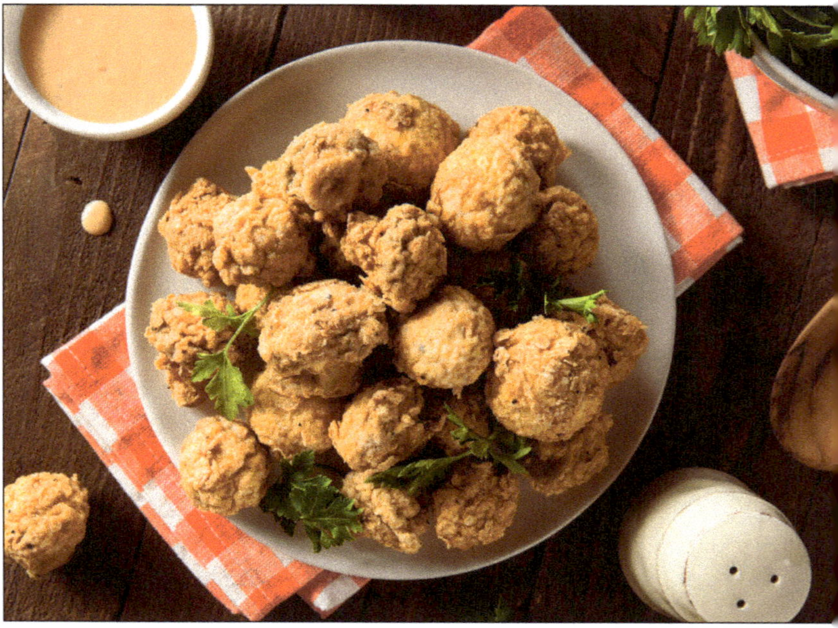

ingredients

14 mushrooms, Cremini or Baby Bella

1 C panko breadcrumbs, more if needed

3 T Parmesan cheese, grated

1 tsp garlic powder

½ tsp dried parsley

salt to taste

1–2 eggs

2 C oil for frying, vegetable or avocado

putting it all together

For BAKED, Repeat steps 1-4. Bake at 400°F for 20 minutes.

step 1: Clean mushrooms. Leave stems on. Most say to brush. My preference is to brush them with water, then dry.

step 2: Combine panko, Parmesan cheese, garlic powder, parsley, and salt in a medium resealable plastic bag.

step 3: Beat eggs in a large bowl. Add mushrooms and toss until well coated.

step 4: Place a few mushrooms in panko crumb mixture in the bag and shake to coat. Repeat with all.

For FRIED, heat oil in a deep fryer or large saucepan to 375°F.

step 1: Cook mushrooms in hot oil until golden brown, about 5 minutes. Remove to a paper towel-lined plate to cool and drain.

Sauces to include:

Cool Herb Ranch

makes: 1 cup | **prep time:** 10 minutes

½ C sour cream

½ C mayonnaise

1 T fresh dill, chopped

1 T chives, chopped

1 garlic clove, minced

putting it all together

Combine all and refrigerate until ready to serve.

Smoked Paprika Remoulade

makes: 1 cup | **prep time:** 10 minutes

1 C mayonnaise

1 T Dijon mustard

1 T prepared horseradish

1 T sweet pickle relish

1 tsp smoked paprika

½ tsp Worcestershire sauce

1 tsp hot sauce

1 lemon, squeezed

1 garlic clove, minced

salt and freshly ground black pepper, to taste

putting it all together

Combine all and refrigerate until ready to serve.

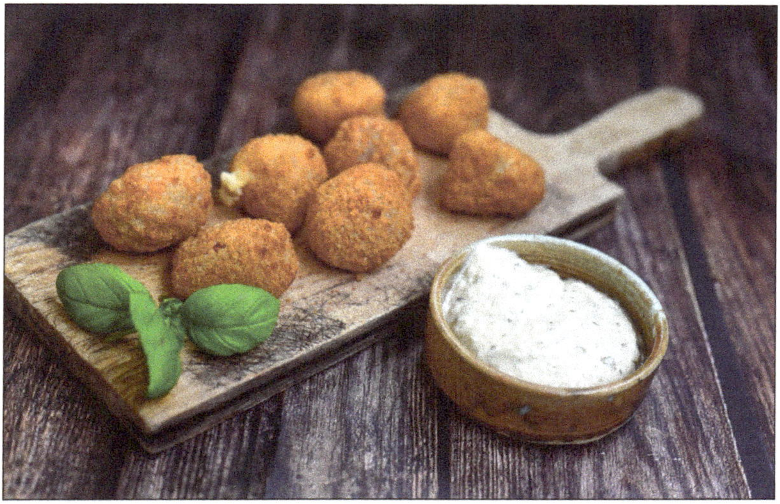

Parmesan Poppers that POP!

This one is for those who love the "popper" taste and pop, but with a cream cheese twist. Oh, there's a kiss of cayenne pepper mixed in, but I'm bypassing the jalapeño bits. The creaminess comes from cream cheese. The dough is simply egg whites and oodles of Parmesan cheese and the kiss of cayenne. A quick fry and these poppers and a favorite sauce will make your tastebuds pop! Serve along with **Cucumber Dipping Sauce** *(recipe follows) while warm.*

makes: 16 Poppers | **prep time:** 20 minutes
cooking time: 20 minutes

ingredients

4 egg whites

8 oz cream cheese, softened

¼ tsp cayenne pepper

2 C Parmesan cheese, grated

1–2 inches of vegetable oil in a small nonstick skillet

putting it all together

step 1: For the dough: whip the egg whites to stiff peaks. Fold in the Parmesan cheese and cayenne pepper.

step 2: For the poppers, flatten one tablespoon of the dough in your hand. Add in ONE tablespoon of softened cream cheese in the center. Create a ball around the cream cheese with dough—pinch closed. Repeat until all dough is used up.

step 3: Heat the vegetable oil to medium-high. Fry until golden, turning once—around ONE minute. Remove from oil, drain, and serve warm. To add a bit more cheese, roll or sprinkle additional Parmesan cheese on each popper.

Cucumber Dipping Sauce

makes: 1½ cups | **prep time:** 15 minutes

ingredients

1 C Greek yogurt

1 C cucumber, seedless, finely chopped-not peeled

1 T lemon juice

1 green onion, finely chopped

½ C basil, chopped

½ tsp garlic powder

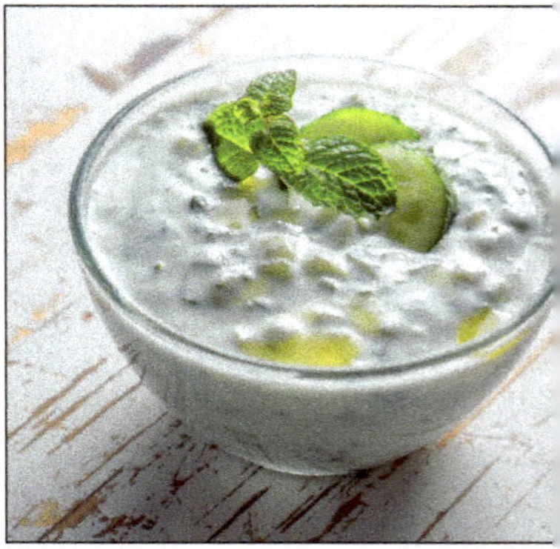

putting it all together

Peel, chop, and mince. Stir all together and refrigerate until ready to serve.

Spinach Bites with Pine Nuts

The pine nuts and nutmeg in the Spinach Bites are always a pleasant surprise. The cheese adds a creamy texture, spinach has a sense of health, and the eggs do the binding for you.

makes: 12 to 15 Bites | **preheat:** oven to 400°F
prep time: 10 minutes | **cooking time:** less than 15 minutes

ingredients

10–12 oz cleaned raw baby spinach or frozen

⅔ C cottage cheese or ricotta cheese

2 eggs

pepper to taste

garlic to taste

1 tsp nutmeg

¾ C pine nuts

Parmesan cheese, grated, to sprinkle on top

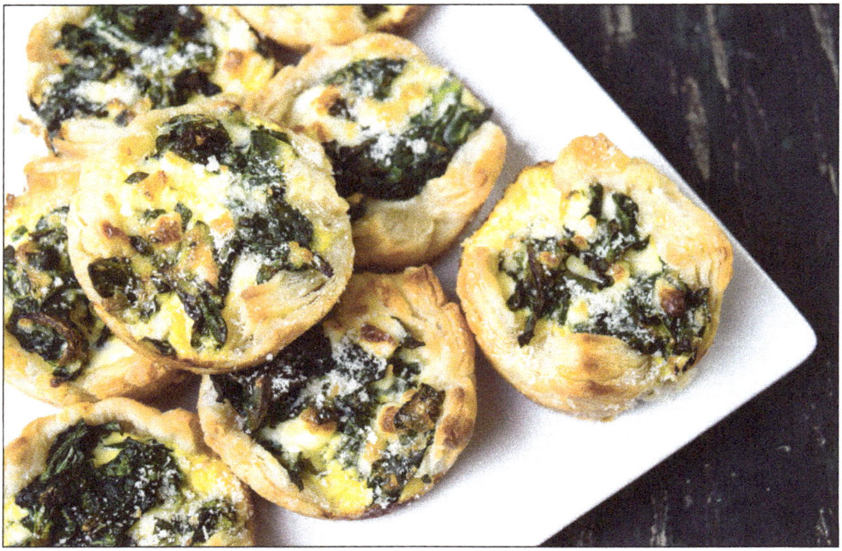

putting it all together

step 1: Clean spinach. If using frozen, thaw. Squeeze with your hands, then drain. Squeeze again, drain.

step 2: Roast pine nuts in a dry pan over medium heat on stovetop for about 4-5 minutes until golden brown. Stay close. They can burn quickly.

step 3: Pulse spinach in food processor or put in blender if you don't have one.

step 4: In a bowl, combine the eggs, garlic, pepper, nutmeg, and mix. Add this mixture into the spinach. Pulse again.

step 5: Use nonstick spray on a mini muffin pan and fill with mixture; top with Parmesan cheese to your taste and roasted pine nuts. Bake.

Remove from mini muffin pan and let stand about 5 minutes, then serve.

Squashed Potatoes

Think of this as finger food potatoes that aren't French Fries ... a step up—although forks are welcome! It's a different type of appetizer that will surprise your guests. The small creamy potatoes in grocery stores that are a large walnut size are your starting point. I get them in Costco's veggie area. Precooking them, you will then add another layer of cooking to crisp up, then provide a few dipping sauces of your choice. Sour cream and **chili lime aioli** *(recipe follows) are my favorites for this appetizer.*

makes: 8 to 10 squashed potatoes

prep time and cooking time: less than 30 minutes for both stages

ingredients

1 lb of Yukon Golds, small, walnut-size—*also known as creamy potatoes*

4 T butter

½ C sour cream

4 chives, chopped

sea salt and pepper to taste

Options: add on other sauces and toppings of choice

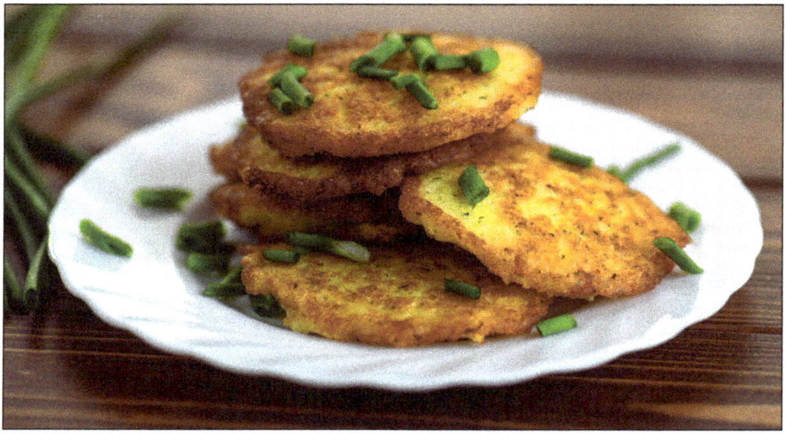

putting it all together

step 1: Place unpeeled potatoes in a large pot, cover with cold water, add salt. Bring them to a boil for 15-20 minutes. Drain.

step 2: Squash each potato. Using the base of a sturdy drinking glass or measuring cup, squash the potatoes until creamy—a few lumps are welcomed.

step 3: Melt butter in a fry pan and cook each side of the squashed potatoes to a golden brown. Drain on paper towel … serve warm with chives, sour cream, or other toppings of choice.

Favorite sauces: sour cream, **Chili Lime Aioli,** page 112, and/or jalapeño cream.

Chewy facts about potatoes ...

Vincent Van Gough painted four still-life paintings featuring potatoes.

Potatoes didn't arrive in Idaho until 1836.

During the gold rush, potatoes were highly valued. At a time when gold was more plentiful than nutrition sources, you might say that potatoes were worth their weight in gold!

Potatoes are a vitamin C source: 45 % of daily require can come from just one medium spud!

In 1903, Parker Brothers had a game called "The Potato Race."

Potatoes were the first vegetable grown in space in 1995.

Potato is the 4th most important crop worldwide.

35% of the potato crop is turned into french fries, 28% is used for fresh, and 13% goes to chips!

On average, US residents consume 110 pounds of potatoes per year. Europeans consume twice that much!

A potato has more potassium than a banana!

August 13 is National Potato Day, don't forget to celebrate!

Sweet Chili Cheesy Stuffed Mushrooms

One of the easiest appetizers to whip up is a stuffed mushroom. This one was a "concoction" that came together when I had extra Baby Bella mushrooms. Opening the refrigerator, I pulled out cottage cheese, cheddar cheese, and Boursin cheese. Mixing them together, I added a kiss of garlic salt and reached for the Sweet Chili Sauce. Delicious.

makes: enough to stuff 30 mushrooms | **preheat:** oven to 350°F
prep time: 20 minutes | **cooking time:** 15-20 minutes

ingredients

Baby Bella, Cremini or White Oyster mushrooms

1 package of Boursin cheese—*I use herbs and chives*

8 oz cottage cheese, regular or small curd

¾ C cheddar cheese

¼ C sweet chili sauce

garlic salt to taste

putting it all together

step 1: Clean mushrooms and remove stems. Don't soak mushrooms, they will instantly absorb water. Rinse off and dry before stuffing.

step 2: Mix all other ingredients together and spoon generously into mushrooms.

step 3: Place on a baking sheet or open baking dish and cook until mushrooms feel soft to the touch—they are done.

Serve immediately.

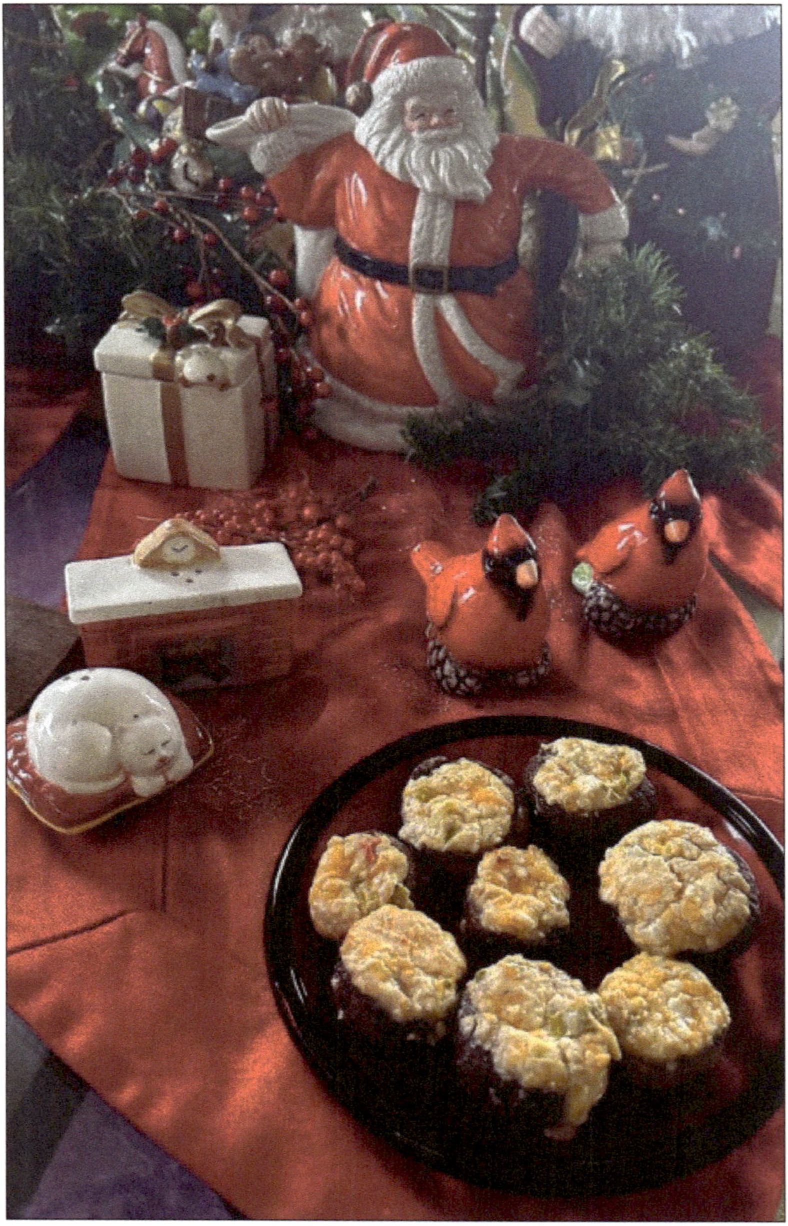

Sweet Chili Cheesy Stuffed Mushrooms

Yellow Zucchini Soup Sippers

Many times, I will have soup sippers as part of my appetizer offerings. When I do this, there is at least one nibble along with the sipping one. Think asparagus, mushroom, zucchini, even a cheesy soup that might be delicious to have in a small proportion as a "tease" versus the full mug or bowl.

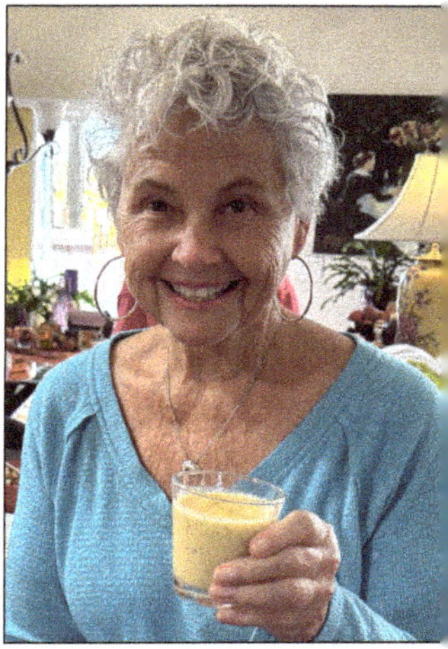

Sometimes, when I have my Second Saturday Author Gatherings in my home, I will have a pot of soup I had made early that morning. On my kitchen island, I will bring the pot out, at least a dozen small pudding-sized glasses or ceramics. Always a hit, part of my appetizer repertoire as well.

makes: 15, 4- to 6-oz mini glasses
prep time: 30 minutes | **cooking time:** 30 minutes

ingredients

1 onion, Maui, Vidalia, or white, chopped

2 T butter

4 yellow zucchini, diced into large slices or chunks

6 C chicken broth—*I prefer Better than Bouillon*

1 russet potato, peeled and diced into large slices or chunks

¾ C cheddar cheese, grated

3 chives or green onions, greens only, chopped

salt & pepper to taste

putting it all together

step 1: Dice onions and sauté in butter. Add cut-up zucchini and broth. Add peeled, cut-up potato, which is used for thickening and adding flavor. Simmer until tender. Add cheese, blending in until melted.

step 2: Remove from the stove ... let cool, then add a few cups at a time to your blender and blend. After all is blended, add it back to the cooking pot. Season. You may want to add more cheese.

step 3: Serve hot. At serving, add a few chopped chives to each serving glass/cup. I usually include teaspoons with servings. Guests have a choice to sip or spoon the zucchini soup.

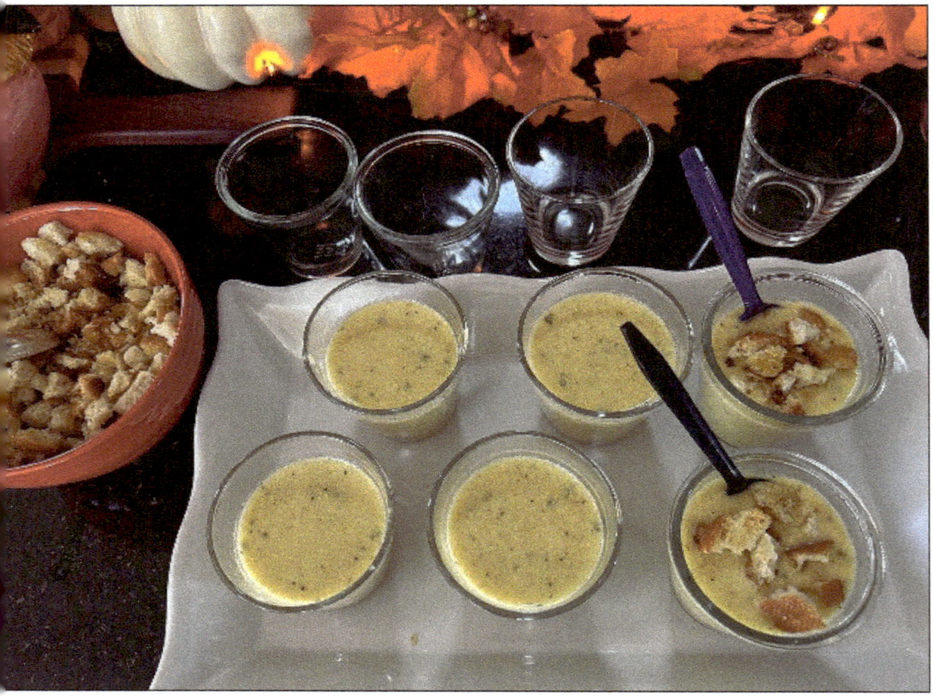

Zesty Red Peppers Bruschetta

Give me a jar of red peppers, and it will disappear fast. If I have several fresh red peppers, I roast them until they blister in the oven for peeling. Combine with basil, cheeses, maybe a little pesto (sometimes lots), definitely garlic, and who knows what else. Add it to a toasted baguette, and it becomes a meal for me. Hello, bruschetta land!

The sweetness of the peppers with the garlic and fresh basil can't be beat. During the summer months, this is a huge ask from friends when we gather on my deck. With a beverage of choice ... foodie and tasty heaven!

makes: 20 bruschetta | **preheat:** oven to 400°F
prep and cooking time: 45–60 minutes

ingredients

2 medium sweet red peppers, halved and seeded
OR a jar of roasted red peppers

1 whole garlic bulb—*all the cloves*

1 tsp plus 2 T olive oil, divided

3 T fresh parsley, minced

3 T fresh basil, minced **OR** 2 tsp dried basil

1 T lemon juice

½ tsp salt

¼ tsp pepper

1 baguette, sliced

Extra olive oil for sprinkling on top—*if you don't use the jarred red peppers*

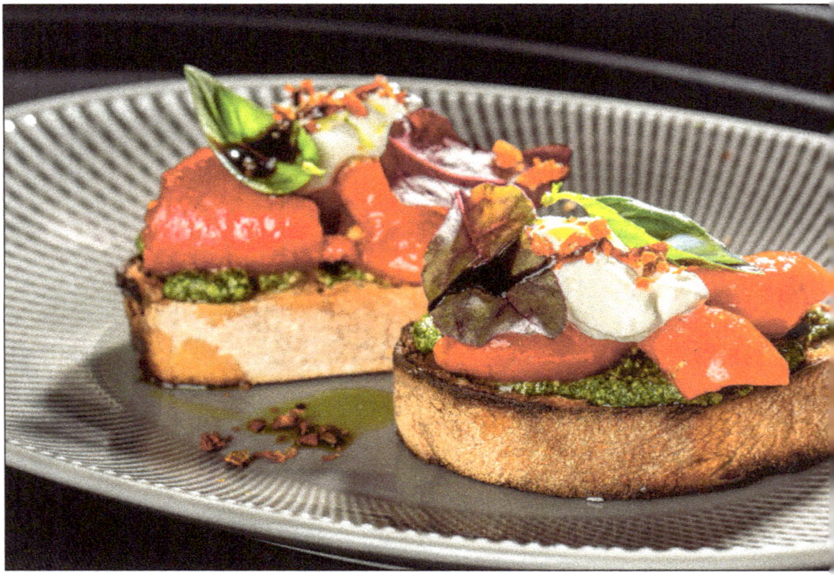

putting it all together

step 1: Remove papery outer skin from garlic bulb—do not fully peel or separate cloves. Brush with 1 teaspoon of olive oil. Wrap in heavy-duty foil. Roast until softened, about 45 minutes in 400° F oven. Cool.

step 2: If not using jarred peppers, broil fresh red peppers 4 inches from the heat until skins blister, about 10 minutes. Immediately place peppers in a bowl; cover with plastic wrap and let stand for 15-20 minutes.

step 3: Peel off and discard charred skin from garlic. Cut the top off of garlic head, leaving root end intact. Squeeze softened garlic the from bulb and finely chop. Coarsely chop peppers.

step 4: In a bowl, combine the parsley, basil, lemon juice, salt, pepper, and remaining oil. Add peppers and garlic; mix well.

step 5: Cut bread into 16 slices, ½-inch thick; broil until lightly toasted. Top with pepper mixture. Serve immediately.

Cheesy Mushroom Crostini

As I wrote this up, my taste buds and mouth were telling me to go make it right away. What's great about mushrooms ,as they gently cook in a buttery garlic, or merge with ingredients that land in the oven, is the promise of a great taste sensation when the finished treat lands in my mouth. After all, the cook should be sampling, yes?

What I love about mushroom appetizers is that they offer a creamy texture along with mushroom bites woven with cheese. The result is a rich taste. Partial comfort with an elegant side to them.

makes: 20 crostini | **preheat:** oven to 375°F
prep time: 20 minutes | **cooking time:** about 4–5 minutes, until cheese bubbles

ingredients

1 baguette, sliced ⅜- to ½ -inch thick

1 lb seasonal mushrooms, Shiitakes, Baby Bellas, Creminis, Chanterelles, even Shitakes

1 shallot, minced

1 tsp garlic powder

2 T butter

1 C smoked cheese, grated

½ C mayonnaise or sour cream

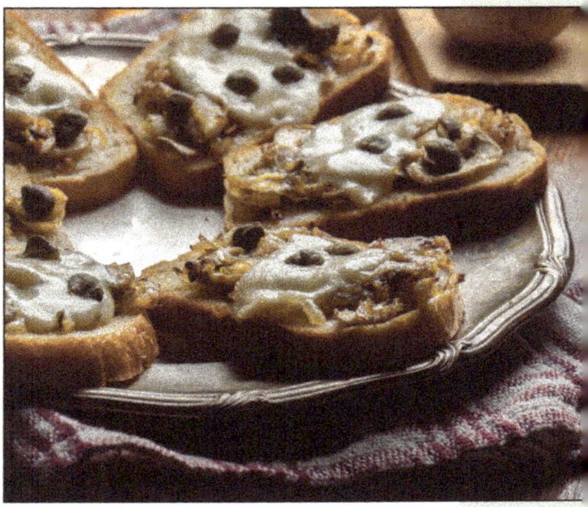

putting it all together

step 1: Brush/clean mushrooms, trim stems.

step 2: Sauté mushrooms, shallot, and garlic in butter.

step 3: Mix in cheese and mayonnaise or sour cream.

step 4: Spread the mixture generously over baguette slices and bake until the cheese bubbles and edges are golden.

Mediterranean Veggie Crostini

Warm weather brings together so many things I love about crostini —pesto, pine nuts, basil, cheese, Kalamata olives, and the variety of fresh vegetables that are easily available to chop, dice, and mince away. With the first bite, my guests reach for another crostini for their appetizer plate! You can make your pesto from scratch. I no longer do—the jarred basil pesto in the refrigerated deli section of Costco is one of the best I've had. Do the cheat and just get it. The rest of the crostini comes together quickly and I promise—it will be a star of your offerings.

makes: 35 crostini | **preheat:** oven to 400°F to 450°F
prep time: 20 minutes | **cooking time:** 55 minutes

ingredients

2 baguettes, sliced in ¼-inch pieces

½ C pine nuts

¾ basil leaves, off stems

1 C basil pesto—*I love the Costco pesto!*

1 C mozzarella cheese, shredded

1 C Kalamata olives, pitted, cut in half

1 bell pepper, halved and seeded

½ eggplant, thinly sliced

1 zucchini, thinly sliced

½ red onion, peeled and thinly chopped

olive oil

option: French's Fried Onions

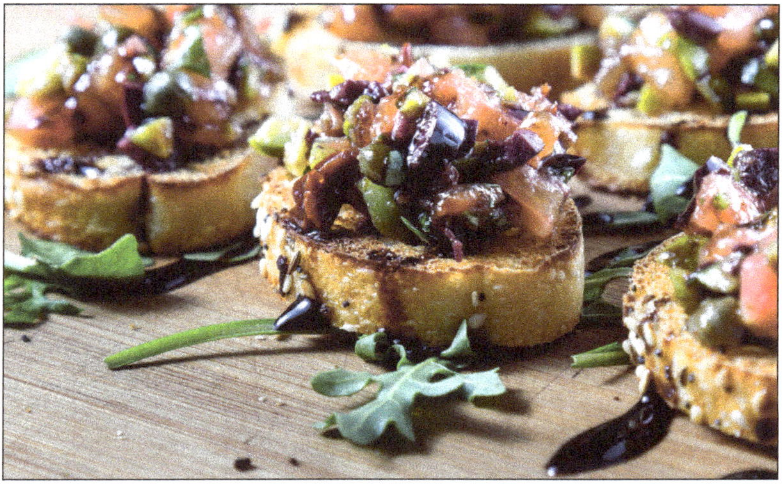

putting it all together

step 1: With the two baguettes, slice and make **Crostini** recipe on page 45.

step 2: With a dry pan/skillet, add the pine nuts and toast lightly over a low to medium heat for just a few minutes—you want a touch of golden brown. Shake the pan to distribute the heat. Set aside.

step 3: Preheat oven to 400°F–450°F for 30 to 40 minutes. Rub the bell pepper with olive oil, cut in half lengthwise, remove seeds and white pith, and place cut-side down down on a parchment-lined baking sheet. Roast until the skins are deeply wrinkled and charred. Remove from oven; wrap in foil. When cool, the peeling is easy. Slice the pepper into thin strips.

step 4: Add chopped red onion to pesto.

step 5: Cut eggplant, red pepper, and zucchini in half. Brush with olive oil. Broil each side for 2 minutes.

step 6: Shred or slice the mozzarella into small pieces or thin slices.

step 7: Start your assembly: crostini, pesto, mozzarella, veggies, topped with sliced Kalamata olives, a few pine nuts, and basil leaves. Add a few French's Fried Onions on top for an added bite crunch.

Sweet Potato Crostini

If you are looking for a crostini-type of appetizer without the bread, the Sweet Potato Crostini may be your answer. It's low-carb and gluten-free. In place of bread, you get sweet potato baked rounds with warmed brie, pecans, and cranberries. If nuts are a problem, eliminate the pecans.

makes: 25 crostini | **preheat:** oven to 400°F
prep time: 20 minutes | **cooking time:** 30 minutes

ingredients

3 medium sweet potatoes, peeled

1 tsp kosher salt

1 tsp black pepper

1 tsp cinnamon

1 T light brown sugar

1 (12 oz) wheel Brie, cut into 1-inch slices

¾ C pecans, roughly chopped, toasted

½ C dried cranberries

honey, for drizzling

nonstick olive oil spray

putting it all together

step 1: Preheat oven to 400°F and line a baking sheet with parchment paper. Peel potatoes and slice into ¼ -inch thick pieces.

step 2: In a small bowl, combine the brown sugar, salt, pepper, and cinnamon.

step 3: Spray the sweet potatoes with the nonstick olive oil spray and then sprinkle them with the spice mixture.

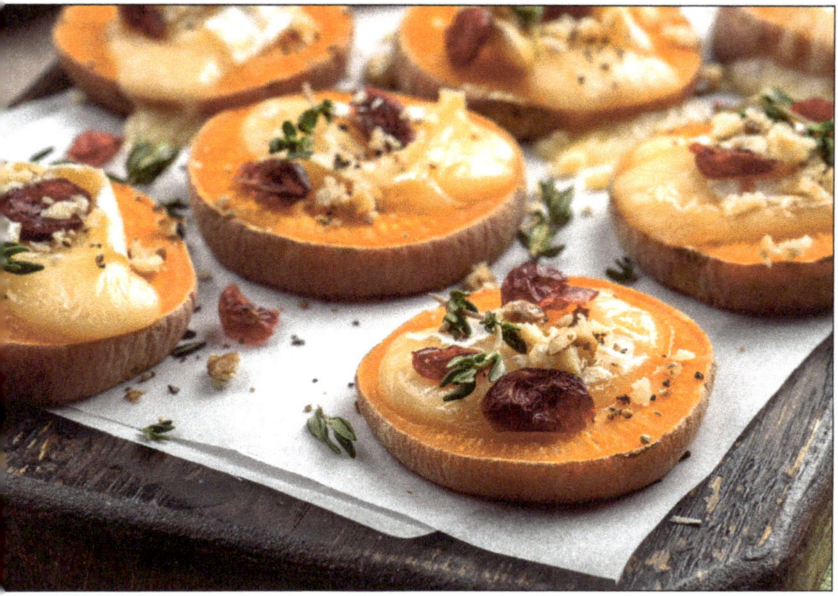

step 4: Roast sweet potato slices until tender, about 25 minutes. Remove to a rack to cool.

step 5: Toast the pecans in a dry skillet on stove top for 3 to 5 minutes. Stir often, no oil needed. Cool, then chop.

step 6: Top baked sweet potato slices with Brie, pecans, and cranberries.

step 7: Bake 5 more minutes or until the Brie is melty. Finish them off with a drizzle of honey.

Serve warm.

Asparagus Brie Puff Pastry Pop Ups

Once springtime hits, the grocery store is alive with asparagus. Thin ones and thick ones and everything in between. You can enjoy them through the summer. Typically, it's served cold after al dente cooking with other veggies on a tray with a dip of some sort. Go beyond the standard veggie and dip spread and the side combos most of us come up with. Why not a hot appetizer that is easy peasy and is a surprise with the soft cheese resting under the asparagus, like a Brie? Adding capers and pine nuts delivered with a kiss of lemon pepper to the mix, creates a winner for your guests.

makes: 1 large tart | **preheat:** oven to 375°F
prep time: 15 minutes | **cooking time:** from 17–20 minutes

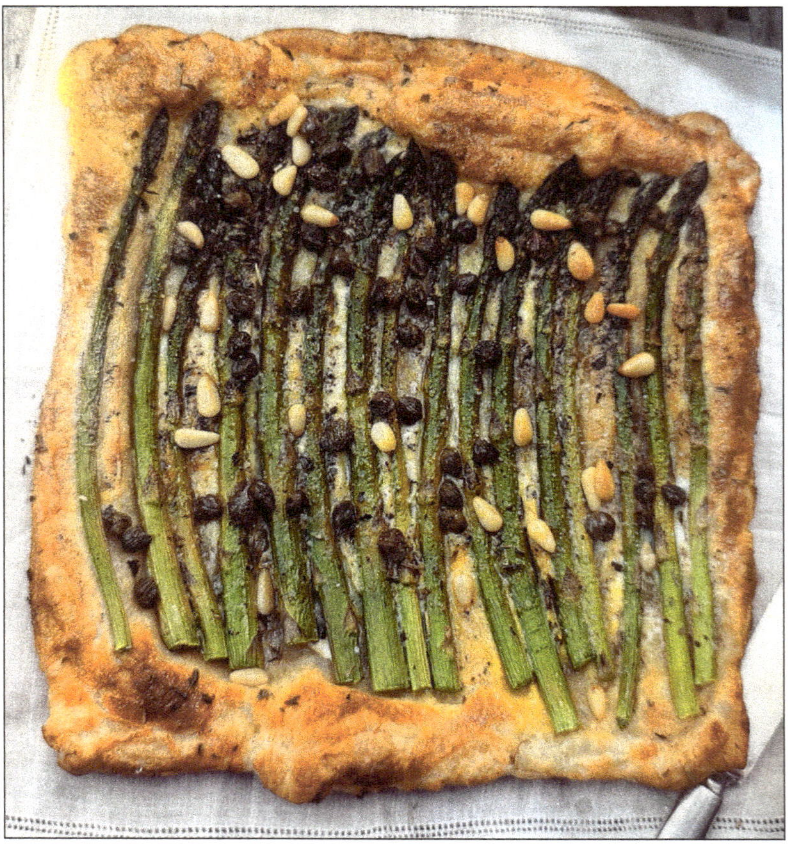

ingredients

1 puff pastry sheet

asparagus, snap the lower section, only tender parts

avocado or olive oil—*very little to sprinkle over puff pastry*

1–2 eggs

Brie cheese, 6-inch, large wedge or small round, rind removed, softened

3 T pine nuts

3 T capers

¾ tsp garlic powder

1 tsp basil leaves, ground

1–2 tsp lemon pepper

putting it all together

step 1: Roll puff pastry on a lightly floured counter—move it to a cookie sheet that has been lightly sprayed with a nonstick cooking spray. Pinch up edges for the crust. Spread a thin layer of the Brie (remove rind) on the pastry. Mix the eggs and brush a thin layer on top of the cheese layer. Make sure you include all edging.

Note: you can precut the puff pastry for mini pieces. Pinch all the edges and complete your "putting it together." Reduce your baking time to 15 minutes.

step 2: Cut asparagus and lay on top of the egg mixture. Add pine nuts, capers, basil, garlic, and lemon pepper.

step 3: Bake. You want your puff pastry to be golden brown.

step 4: As it cools, cut into serving pieces.

Feta and Zucchini Puffs with Pine Nuts

This easy appetizer recipe is great for quick entertaining. The feta cheese adds a light and creamy bite to the rich, sautéed zucchini and cheese-filled cups that will make friends want another. I always think of pine nuts as one of the "treasures" from Nutland to enjoy. They add visual promise of added tastes and nuttiness.

Puffs are easy to pull together and satisfy the taste buds of party goers. The mixture of feta, mayo, and Parmesan create the structure to add the spinach and lemon for a healthier feel.

makes: 24 puff pastry bites | **preheat:** oven to 375°F
prep time: 15 minutes | **cooking time:** 14 minutes
Cool for a few minutes before serving

ingredients

1 sheet frozen puff pastry, thawed in the refrigerator

¾ C mayonnaise

10 oz feta cheese—*get fresh feta, then crumble it*

½ C freshly grated Parmesan cheese

1 yellow zucchini, thinly sliced

1 green zucchini, thinly sliced

2 garlic cloves, minced

1 lemon, zest half … add 1 tsp juice

½ tsp ground black pepper

1 C pine nuts

putting it all together

step 1: Spray a 24-cup mini muffin pan or two 12-cup mini muffin pans with nonstick cooking spray.

step 2: Roll out the thawed but cold puff pastry sheet on a lightly floured surface into a rectangle using a rolling pin. Cut into 24 (approximately 2½-inch) squares. Lightly press puff pastry squares into each cup of the prepared mini muffin pan, and prick with a fork.

step 3: Roast pine nuts in a dry pan over a medium heat. Stir often for about 4-5 minutes until they are golden brown and fragrant. Stay close, they can burn quickly. Put aside … you will top each puff with several pine nuts before baking.

step 4: Mix the mayonnaise, feta cheese, Parmesan cheese, spinach, garlic, and pepper in a bowl. Thinly slice the zucchinis, chop, and add to mixture.

step 5: Scoop zucchini mixture evenly into the cups—about ¾ full. Add several pine nuts on top, poking a few within the mix.

step 6: Bake in the preheated oven until pastry is puffed and the corners are golden brown, 14-15 minutes.

step 7: Cool in the pan on a wire rack for 5 minutes before transferring the bites to a serving dish.

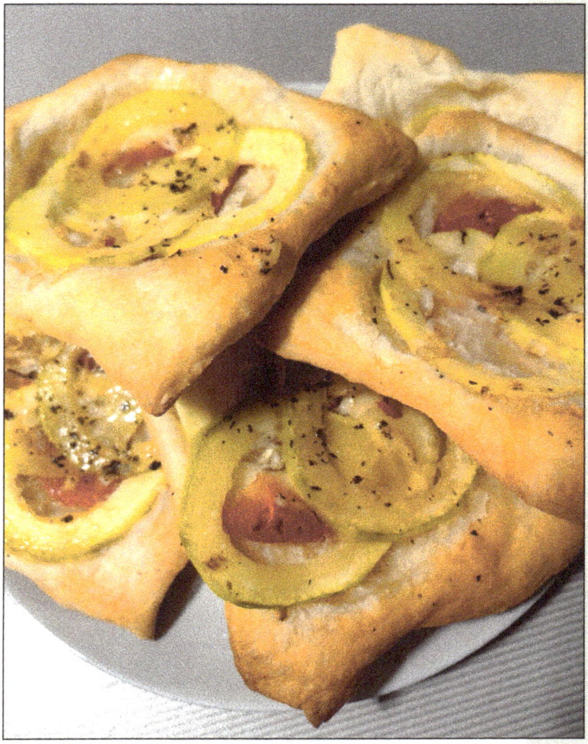

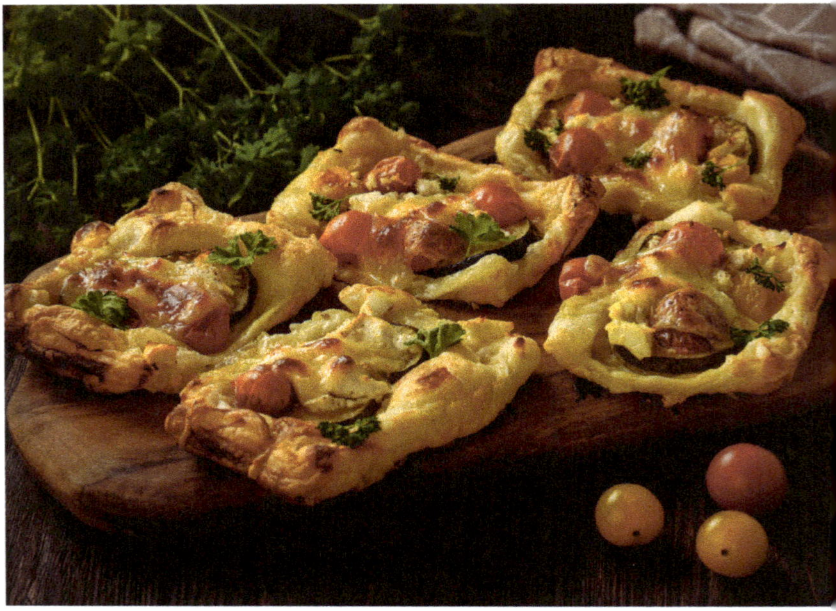

Zucchini Puff Pastry Pop Ups

Zucchini is available year round in most places. For gardeners, the lookout for ways to use the abundant vegetable becomes a quest. Go beyond the standard veggie and dip spread and the side combos most of us come up with. Why not a hot appetizer that is easy peasy and is a welcomed "add" to the close-by raw veggie platter, especially in the summer months? Cheeses, garlic, eggs, and nuts all come into my "Let's do this fast and a tad different?" Maybe grape tomatoes to add to the mix. I usually have puff pastry in my freezer, and I'm ready to put it all together.

makes: 16 to 20 depending on cutting size | **preheat:** oven to 375°F
prep time: 30 minutes | **cooking time:** 16–20 minutes.

ingredients

2 pasty pastry sheets, thawed

1 each yellow and green zucchini, thinly sliced

avocado or olive oil—*very little to sprinkle over puff pastry*

1–2 eggs

1½ C feta or Brie cheese

1 C grape or cherry tomatoes, sliced or cut

1 C basil leaves, cut

putting it together

step 1: Slice zucchini and spread out on paper towels to let it "weep" a bit so your slices have less moisture.

step 2: Puff pastry at room temp. With a little flour, roll to thin, then pinch up edges on all sides. On a large cookie sheet, move your pastry and sprinkle olive oil and spread lightly with your fingers or brush. Mix eggs and brush over the entire surface of the puff pastry. Spread zucchini slices, feta, or Brie cheese *(be generous here)* that has been crumpled up over the surface. Add your tomato.

step 3: Sprinkle with garlic and some of the cut up basil leaves—*I usually roll several leaves, then slice thinly in ribbons with a knife.*

step 4: Bake for 16 to 20 minutes at 375 F. You want your puff pastry to become golden brown.

step 5: As it cools, cut into serving pieces, add a fresh leaf of basil to each slice.

Cooking from your heart

welcomes new and old friends ...

a perfect gathering in the making!

— Judith Briles

Cheese … Cheese … Cheese

Cheese appetizers offer a range of flavors and textures, from classic dips to elegant baked options. I always have a few for party gatherings … but sometimes, when it's a "not cook day" a plate of crackers, breads, and cheeses becomes my perfecto meal. The best choice often depends on the occasion and personal preference. *Think creamy dips, baked brie, even cheese balls.*

For stuffing appetizers with cheese, I've used many kinds—from cottage cheese that I add to stuffed mushrooms with a cheddar and chili sauce, to the variety of bleu cheeses. Sometimes adding sour cream or cream cheese to the mix works well with a firm cheese. I'm a bleu cheese kind of gal and have always loved the tangy flavor that fills my mouth with that first taste. You can go from mild to bold. Piping may be an option, although it's one I don't use—I like the feel of using my hands.

What I love about bleu cheeses is that they are great mixers—whether with nuts or fruit like pears, apples, and figs, and of course, savory partners—think olives, mushrooms, celery, even shrimp.

Do yourself, your guests, and your tastebuds a favor and avoid any pre-crumbled bleu cheese. Stick with a wedge, and break it up as you use.

Serving temp is up to you. Sometimes chilled, warmed, or room temperature. Room temp is often the landing spot—if they should be chilled, chilled platters and serving dishes on ice work. Warm/hot should have a heating element beneath them. Your recipe should be the guide.

My Favorite Mild and Creamy Bleu Cheeses

These blend with cream cheese or sour cream and are not overwhelming.

Gorgonzola Dolce: A sweet and ultra-creamy Italian bleu cheese, excellent for spreading or mixing into fillings.

Danish Bleu (Danablu): Known for being rich and creamy with a slightly more mellow, savory flavor compared to stronger bleus.

Cambozola: A German cheese that combines the creaminess of Camembert with a hint of bleu mold, resulting in a very mild, buttery flavor.

Bold and Strong Bleu Cheeses

Think power robust tasting—these partner well with nuts, bacon, even a kiss of amaretto, bourbon, brandy, or rum.

Roquefort: A French sheep's milk cheese with a distinct sharp, tangy, and sometimes "stinky" flavor. When I have a good roquefort, just a slice is enough … or a cracker to hold it as I nibble through it.

Stilton: A classic English bleu cheese that is rich, savory, and fudge-like, often paired with after dinner drinks.

Maytag Bleu: An American classic with a creamy yet crumbly texture and bold, lemony, pungent notes.

Think Cheesy Appetizers

Spinach Artichoke Dip: A perennial favorite, this warm, creamy dip combines earthy spinach, tangy artichoke hearts, and rich cheese for a satisfying starter.

Baked Brie: This elegant appetizer is simple to prepare. Brie is baked until gooey, often topped with fig preserves, jams, cranberry sauce, or nuts, and served with crackers or bread. I love to split a brie, stuff with nuts and jam, and wrap in pastry (do the splitting with dental floss)—bake so that the cheese oozes when cut. And definitely add some to the inner filling to the top at presentation. This makes me hungry as I write it.

Charcuterie Board: While a board often features meats and fruits, cheese is the usual star. Offering a variety of hard (aged cheddar, Parmesan), semi-soft (Gouda, Havarti are favorites), and soft cheeses (Brie, goat cheese) ensures that your nibblers will partake quickly.

Cheese Balls: Versatile and easy to make ahead, cheese balls can be simple or feature additions like bacon, herbs, or pimiento cheese. Think seasons and add fun coloring to the mix.

Queso Dip: A warm, spicy favorite, queso dip is a two-ingredient, slow-cooker option that is easy to make and always a hit with tortilla chips. I like to make my own tortilla chips when I have a small group arriving, versus a big bag from the store.

Goat Cheese or Whipped Feta: For a lighter, fresher option, a whipped dip with hot honey, lemon, or roasted nuts provides a unique sweet and savory flavor profile. Adding large olives to the mix is welcomed. And strong suggestion: if you have a Middle Eastern small grocery close by, visit it.

Often, there are a variety of fetas—Hungarian, Bulgarian, French, etc. So much tastier that the drier American counterpart—and definitely creamier. I've made appetizer plates with three—drizzle olive oil on fetas, add multiple olives, dried apricots and a sliced baguette. A personal favorite of mine.

putting it all together

Variety is always welcomed: Mix it up. Soft, hard, and crumble. Mild, Sharp.

Temperature counts: Most cheeses taste best when served at room temperature, so allow them to sit out for a bit before the party starts.

Pairings: Serve cheeses with a variety of accompaniments like crackers, bread, fruit, nuts, and chutneys to enhance the flavors.

There are three possible parts to a date,
of which at least two must be offered:
entertainment, food, and affection.
It is customary to begin a series of dates
with a great deal of entertainment,
a moderate amount of food,
and the merest suggestion of affection.
As the amount of affection increases,
the entertainment can be reduced proportionately.
When the affection IS the entertainment,
we no longer call it dating.
Under no circumstances can the food be omitted.

— Judith Martin, Miss Manners

Essentials for Judith's Kitchen

Most of my pots and pans are on a large rack hung from the ceiling. My knives are not put away. I have two magnetic racks that their blades attach to. And I have three containers that I keep extra "tasting/stirring" spoons in. Two are on each side of the stove top. One rests by a larger container full of wood spoons of all sizes and cooking utensils. The third is on another counter I call the "drinks bar"—coffee, tea, and wine. All I need to do is reach and use.

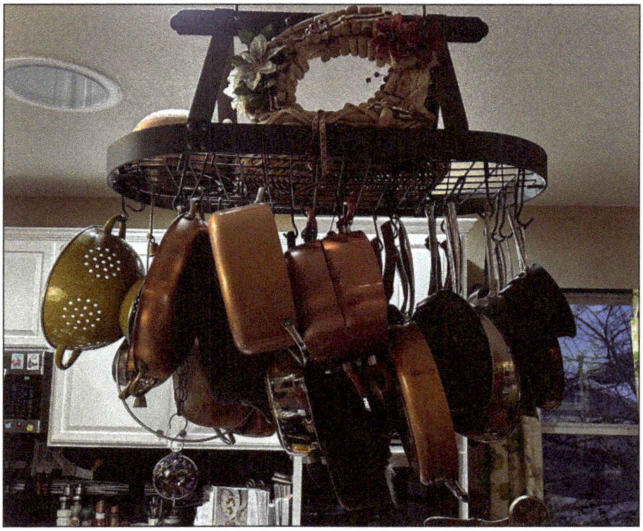

My kitchen sink has two musts for me: an instant "hot" dispenser, perfect for a mug of tea **AND** a faucet that I can touch with a finger to turn on or off—sometimes a forearm if my hands are floured or full of mixing something.

When space is limited, finding ways to use stackable racks and shelves delivers more options. I have two pantries. One in the main kitchen that is used daily / weekly. The other is in the garage—backups and to resupply the kitchen. Its companions are a refrigerator that is an overflow backup, especially when we have house guests or are entertaining, and a separate freezer.

PANTRY

Almond milk, boxed

Albacore tuna

Anchovies

Artichoke hearts

Avocado oil

Beans: black, refried, cannellini

Beets: pickled, sliced

Capers

Chestnuts

Corn: whole and creamed

Chili sauce: Thai sweet

Chipotle peppers in adobo sauce

Chocolate chips

Cornmeal

Crackers, various: Ritz, Butter, Wheat, Artisan

Dates, Medjool

Fruit, dried: apricots, figs, cherries, cranberries, raisins

Garlic: whole heads, ground and minced in jars

Honey: jarred and powder

Hot Sauce: Cholula, Tabasco, Sriracha

Jams and Jellies: apricot, marionberry, grape, blackberry, mint, cran peño, sweet heat … *just keep the ones you want … give away or toss all others.*

Juices: apple and peach mango

Lentils

Maple syrup—*Costco has one of the best*

Mayonnaise

Marinara (Rao's) and fettuccine sauces

Milk: almond, cashew, evaporated, sweetened condensed

Mushrooms, sliced and bits

Mustards: Dijon, honey, French's yellow, horseradish, ground

Nuts: cashews, pecans, macadamia, pistachios—*for toasting, chopping, and munching*

Oatmeal: regular and instant

Oils: olive oil, extra virgin, avocado, canola, vegetable, garlic from farmer's market

Olives: pimiento-stuffed, garlic-stuffed, black, green, Kalamata

Ortega diced chilis

Panko breadcrumbs

Parmesan cheese, gated

Pastas, dried: wide and narrow noodles, macaroni, spaghetti, linguine, rotini

Peanut butter, jarred and powder

Peppers, jarred and mild: banana rings, red roasted, jalapeño

Pickles: stackers, relish, cornichons (mini), baby dill, red onion

Popcorn, loose kernels, not microwave

Potatoes: russet, Yukon golds, reds

Protein drinks

Red peppers, roasted

Rice: long grain, brown, Arborio, Ben's Original

Salsas: red and verde

Sauces: *Knorr has a variety. Bearnaise is excellent.*

Seasonings, herbs and spices: list out what you use. My opened pantry door has a rack with eight shelves packed larger sizes and a kitchen pull out drawer dedicated to smaller jars. In the summer when I grow basil, dills, and tarragon, leaves are dried and crushed, then jarred and labeled. My small jars come from Ikea. Whatever you use, get labels on lid and/or sides. Once spices pass the one year mark, it's best to replace.

Included are a variety of salts and peppers, curry, chili powder, paprikas, Hatch's green chili powder, cinnamon, onion powder, onion-dried and chopped, Trader Joe's Taco Seasoning. Everything Bagel Seasoning is a good add. Kinders® has a variety I use: lemon pepper, lemon salt, buttery garlic and herb, truffle garlic, Parmesan black garlic.

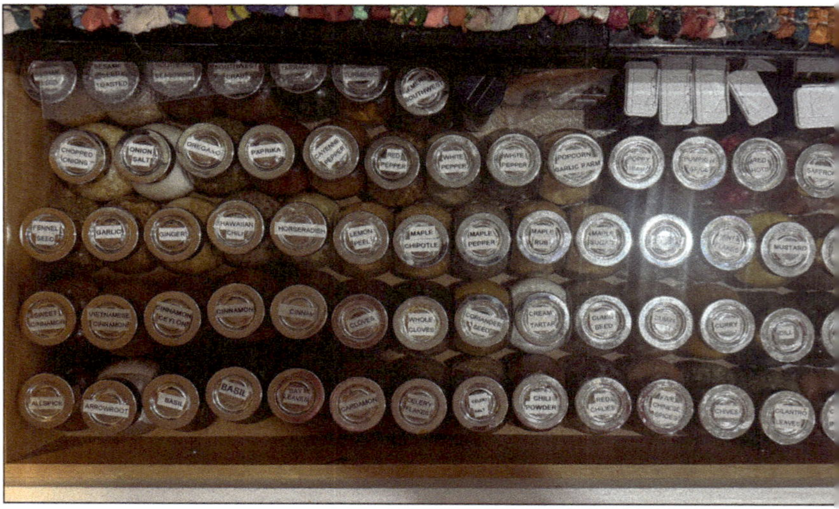

Soups, canned: celery, chicken, mushroom

Sweet Heat—*both jarred and bottled with peppers and jelly*

Broths and stocks, Better Than Bouillon: chicken, beef, vegetable, lobster, sofrito

Teas, various: musts are British and Irish breakfast, Earl Grey, Peach, Crystal Light Peach

Tomatoes: crushed, whole, diced, tomato paste or RO*TEL

Vinegars: apple cider, balsamic, red wine, rice wine, tarragon, white distilled, white wine

BAKING INGREDIENTS

Baking powder

Baking soda

Baking spices: cinnamon, nutmeg, allspice,cloves

Flavored extracts

Flour, all-purpose, bulk

Peppers: coarse, whole, lemon

Salts: kosher, sea, whole, flakes

Sugars: granulated, light and dark brown, powdered

COOKING

Blender

Breville counter stove—*I have a gas stove top and double oven. This is an extra but is often the primary for small cooking/meals.*

Cookie sheets—*I have 10, multiple sizes*

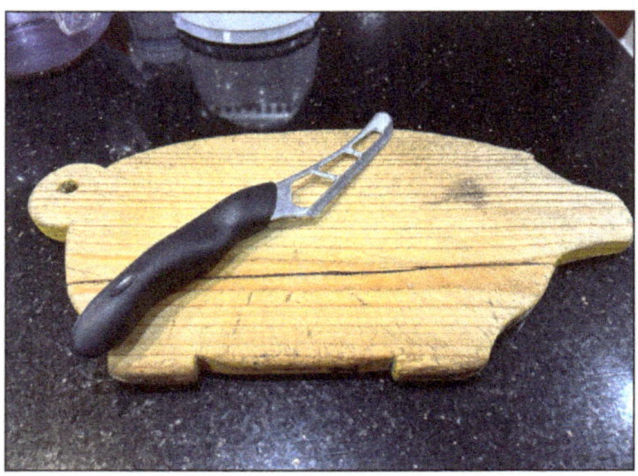

Cutting boards, variety of sizes. *A personal favorite is The Pig … I made him in a woodshop during a summer 70 years ago and he's still in use! I use only wood boards.*

Fish spatula—*I have three of them … most used*

Frying and sauce pans, a variety of sizes: round, square, large, small … many that are used frequently are hung from the ceiling.

Gadgets: zesters, peelers, scoopers, temp gauges, measuring cups (I have quarter to 4 cups), and measuring spoons (several sets)

Hand mixer

Jar Opener—*a must have, I think OXO Good Grips® is one of the best.*

Knives, variety of types—*personal favorite is Cutco cheese and vegetable … the best! I have many paring knives that are used when I have a big prepping to do.*

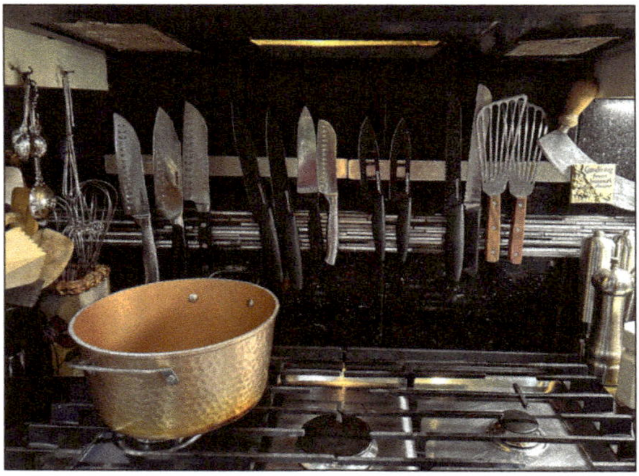

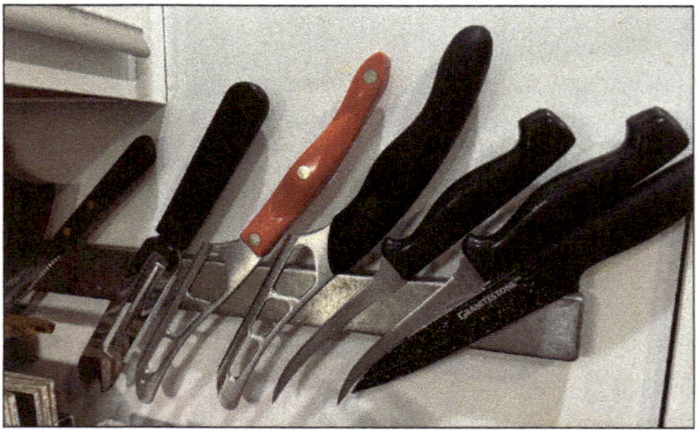

Potholders: *I'm not a user of big and bulky. I have several small ones that I can easily wrap on the ends of whatever is hot.* *Tip*: I keep two small potholders right next to the oven and in the drawer near oven, a large variety.

Pots, several large for soups and large group meals

Roasting pans and racks

Slow cooker, large

Spatulas: several sizes and materials (some suited for hot foods and some for mixing cold)

Wooden utensils: different size spoons, tongs, turners

FRIDGE

Almond milk

Bacon

Basil Pesto

BBQ Sauce—*discover Japanese BBQ*

Beverages: water and juices

Butter, salted and unsalted: Kerrygold Irish is preferred for spreading and toppings; for cooking and baking, I'll use Land O'Lakes or Costco Kirkland.

Cheeses: Boursin, Brie, cheddar, cream, feta, goat, Havarti, pepper jack, Swiss, Velveeta

Cheese, mixed Mexican—*Jack blend that I use for omelets*

Condiments: ketchup, mayonnaise, mustards

Eggs

Fruit, fresh

Squeezes…lemon and lime *for when I don't have fresh*

Vegetables: celery, green onions

Nuts, roasted *to pop into salads*

Tortillas: corn

FREEZER

Beef

Bell Peppers, stuffed from Costco: *excellent and comes with six. I repackage in twos and freeze—a no-thinking meal as an add to salad.*

Baguette and bread loaves, sliced

Chicken: breasts, wings, thighs

Chili, already cooked

Cookies: all kinds that have been baked and can be pulled out for a quick thaw.

Fish: mahi mahi, salmon, sea bass

Fruit: berries and miscellaneous fruits

Nuts: almonds, macadamias, pistachio, pine nuts

Proteins: bacon, hamburger,, ground turkey, fish, shrimp

Puff pastry and pie crusts

Sausage

Soups

In Gratitude ...

Most creatives have others who encourage us, are around us, and look over us to continue to lift and stretch us to do our thing. I'm no different. So many have woven through my life—each makes a difference in so many ways.

My Literary Team

Rebecca Finkel
Peggie Ireland
Mary Salas
Barb Wilson
Nick Zelinger

My Business Team

Leslie Hart
Leah Dasalla
Meg Adverderada
Sheila Mae Mampawa
Sarah Bago
Wubaleme Argogo

My Foodie Friends

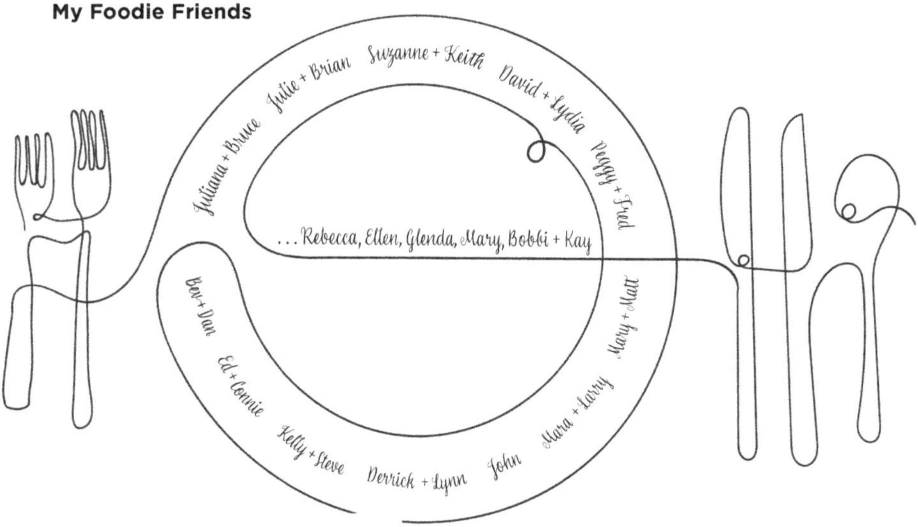

bon appétit

My Neighbor Friends

Cathy Adams
Ron & Melinda Adams
Al Bernier
Ted Gamble
Cindi & Mike Nelson
Jill Taylor & Bob Cartmell
Rita Lucero
Janelle & Gary Mabie
Sandy Kofel
Linda & Ken Nelson
Kathy & Glenn Trice
Rita & Brock Norris
Laura Belsten & Ray Bell
Mindy & Brent Noorgard
Lucy & John Scott

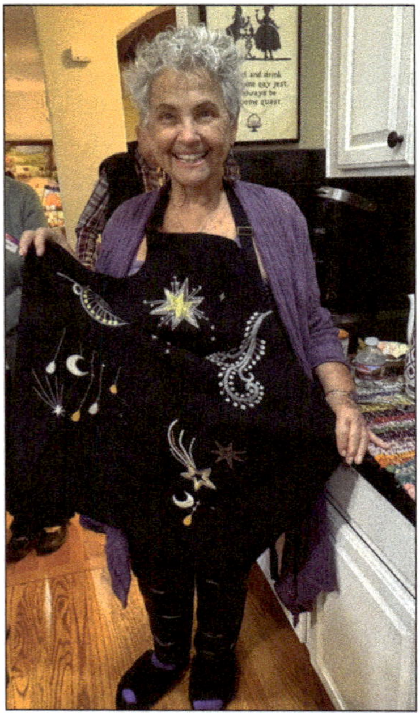

Dr. Judith Briles is the award-winning and bestselling author of 50 books and calls Colorado home. **Appetizers with Judith** joins **Cooking with Judith,** a more general cookbook.

When she's not in the kitchen or in the garden, she's working with clients as **The Book Shepherd,** a book and publishing consulting and project management firm that works with authors at all stages of their book to create and publish a book they never regret! She's the founder of the first Authors Hall of Fame, exclusively dedicated to ensuring the legacy of authors connected in some way with Colorado. Her podcast, **AuthorU-Your Guide to Book Publishing,** is ranked in the top ten in many categories of GoodPods and has had more than 22 million downloads. Judith was honored to be named an Author Laureate by American Book Fest in 2025.

Her publishing and writing titles include *The Author's Walk: Finding and Using Your Voice to Create Publishing Success; How to Avoid Book Publishing Blunders; Author YOU: Creating and Building Your Author and Book Platforms; How to Create Snappy Sassy Salty Success for Authors and Publishers; How to Create CrowdFunding Success for Authors & Writers;* and *How to Create a Million Dollar Speech.*

When God Says NO—Revealing the YES When Adversity and Loss Are Present is her personal memoir, revealing her multiple challenges to climb back when she was knocked down. To date, her books have earned more than 70 book awards.

Judith's historical fiction books written with Brian Barnes include *Book 1: The Secret Journey; Book 2: The Secret Hamlet; Book 3: The Secret Rise;* and *Book 4 :The Secret Awakening.*

Join Judith's Circle for the latest book news: *www.JudithBrilesBooks.com*. Her publishing consulting is at *www.TheBookShepherd.com*.

Judith's
READER CIRCLE

www.JudithBrilesBooks.com

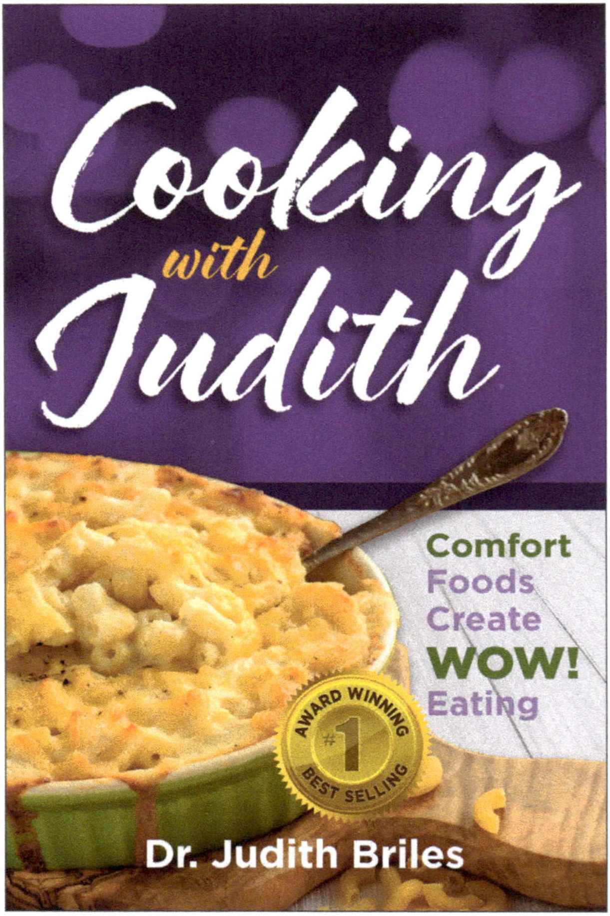

Round out part of your kitchen adventures. Add **Cooking with Judith,** all easy peasy and a welcome add to have fun in the kitchen. You can order online and if your favorite bookstore is sold out, it can easily order it for you.

I've always said that books breed more books. Little did I know that when I published **Cooking with Judith,** there would be a follow-up book. It was obvious it would have to be one on appetizers. It's now in your hands.

A percentage of each booksales is donated to the Rocky Mountain Food Bank.

www.ingramcontent.com/pod-product-compliance
Lightning Source LLC
LaVergne TN
LVHW050912210926
848482LV00012B/409

* 9 7 8 1 8 8 5 3 3 1 1 6 8 *